THE
EVERYTHING
FAMILY NUTRITION

Dear Reader,

Are you ready to take charge of your health? Are you ready to unlock the potential of a nutritious diet? Are you ready to be fit and energetic? If so, you are in the right place.

Every day I hear about the health problems of our nation. We are over-weight and out of shape, and we have more disease and illness than ever before. What's more, we know that diet is the cure for much of what ails us. The key to living a healthy life is no secret. I bet you already have a general idea of changes you could make to improve your overall well-being. But if, like many, you need someone to put it all together for you, you're in luck. This book covers it all, from the basics of nutrition and our diet requirements at every stage of life to delicious recipes and cooking tips to put that knowledge to work for you and your family. Read on to learn about the foods you need and how to incorporate them into an easy, healthy lifestyle designed to maxi-mize nutrition for health and happiness.

Here's to your good health!

Leslie Bilderback

Welcome to the EVERYTHING® Series!

These handy, accessible books give you all you need to tackle a difficult project, gain a new hobby, comprehend a fascinating topic, prepare for an exam, or even brush up on something you learned back in school but have since forgotten.

You can choose to read an *Everything®* book from cover to cover or just pick out the information you want from our four useful boxes: e-questions, e-facts, e-alerts, and e-ssentials.

We give you everything you need to know on the subject, but throw in a lot of fun stuff along the way, too.

We now have more than 400 *Everything®* books in print, spanning such wide-ranging categories as weddings, pregnancy, cooking, music instruction, foreign language, crafts, pets, New Age, and so much more. When you're done reading them all, you can finally say you know *Everything®*!

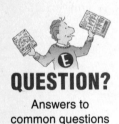

QUESTION?
Answers to
common questions

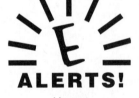

FACTS
Important snippets
of information

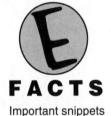

ALERTS!
Urgent
warnings

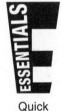

ESSENTIALS
Quick
handy tips

PUBLISHER Karen Cooper

DIRECTOR OF ACQUISITIONS AND INNOVATION Paula Munier

MANAGING EDITOR, EVERYTHING SERIES Lisa Laing

COPY CHIEF Casey Ebert

ACQUISITIONS EDITOR Kerry Smith, Katie McDonough

SENIOR DEVELOPMENT EDITOR Brett Palana-Shanahan

EDITORIAL ASSISTANT Hillary Thompson

Visit the entire Everything® series at *www.everything.com*

THE
EVERYTHING®
FAMILY NUTRITION BOOK

All you need to keep your family
healthy, active, and strong

Leslie Bilderback

Technical Review by Sandra K. Nissenberg, MS, RD

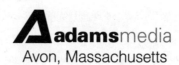

Avon, Massachusetts

For Bill, Emma, and Claire, who are
my motivation for staying healthy.

An Everything® Series Book.
Everything® and everything.com® are registered trademarks of F+W Media, Inc.

Published by Adams Media, a division of F+W Media, Inc.
57 Littlefield Street, Avon, MA 02322. U.S.A.
www.adamsmedia.com

ISBN 10: 1-59869-704-8
ISBN: 13: 978-1-59869-704-9

Printed in the United States of America.

J I H G F E D C B A

Library of Congress Cataloging-in-Publication Data
available from the publisher.

The Everything® Family Nutrition Book is intended as a reference volume only, not as a medical manual. In light of the complex, individual, and specific nature of health problems, this book is not intended to replace professional medical advice. The ideas, procedures, recipes, and suggestions in this book are intended to supplement, not replace, the advice of a trained medical professional. Consult your physician before adopting the suggestions in this book, as well as about any condition that may require diagnosis or medical attention. The authors and publisher disclaim any liability arising directly or indirectly from the use of this book.

This publication is designed to provide accurate and authoritative information with regard to the subject matter covered. It is sold with the understanding that the publisher is not engaged in rendering legal, accounting, or other professional advice. If legal advice or other expert assistance is required, the services of a competent professional person should be sought.
—From a *Declaration of Principles* jointly adopted by a Committee of the American Bar Association and a Committee of Publishers and Associations

Many of the designations used by manufacturers and sellers to distinguish their products are claimed as trademarks. Where those designations appear in this book and Adams Media was aware of a trademark claim, the designations have been printed with initial capital letters.

This book is available at quantity discounts for bulk purchases.
For information, please call 1-800-289-0963.

Contents

Introduction

▶ FOOD IS EVERYWHERE. Every street has a restaurant, every event has a concession stand, and every commercial is dripping with cheese. Billboards, newspapers, and the Internet are constantly trying to sell you food. And you want to buy it. But is what's out there really something you need? Does it do your body any good? Is it making you healthy and strong? And what about the kids? How are they handling being inundated with constant food opportunities? Are they growing up healthy, lean, and fit? If they live in America, there's a good chance they aren't.

Poor nutrition is a growing problem in the United States. It's not that we don't have enough to eat. It's that we have too much of the wrong stuff to eat. You probably already know you should lay off the fast food and pick up an apple instead of that doughnut. But have you ever wondered what healthier foods could really do for you?

Did you know that eating the right carbohydrates can give you ongoing energy? Did you know that bright fruits and vegetables can help protect you against cancer? Did you know that eating right at an early age can protect kids from food allergies? Have you noticed that you feel thirsty after drinking soda, tired after eating cake, and hungry after eating bread? *The Everything® Family Nutrition Book* will shine some light on these subjects and show you exactly what it is you should be eating to help you get the most out of every single day.

Food is fuel. It can be delicious fuel, but it can also be the wrong fuel. Like putting diesel fuel in a gasoline engine, people often choose the wrong food. Without the proper fuel and regular intervals throughout the day, you sputter and stall and will likely need a tuneup, or worse, a complete overhaul. Getting the right fuel is not mysterious, difficult, expensive, or time-consuming. *The Everything® Family Nutrition Book* will show you exactly what, when, and how much you need to eat to get back on the road to good health.

One of the biggest contributors to our poor national diet is our lifestyle. Our hectic families move in multiple directions simultaneously. We rush through or completely skip meals. Exhausted and starving at the end of the day, we are too tired to cook, and so we hit the drive-through on the way home for a bucket, or we meet the kids at the local pizza joint.

We dine out more than the generations that preceded us; so much so that the restaurant business is booming. Sadly, this means that we have forgotten how to cook. What's worse, we aren't teaching our kids to cook. The next generation is coming of age believing that food comes from waiters and cooking is something only TV chefs do.

If we could just get back into the kitchen, cooking our own meals, we could change so much. Not only can it make us healthier, but it will make us happier, too. Spending time in the kitchen doesn't have to be a chore. It can be a warm family time that everyone looks forward to. It can be a time of culinary creativity and experimentation. *The Everything® Family Nutrition Book* will remind you how to cook with delicious, interesting, healthful recipes. It shows how to teach your kids to cook, how to build a nutritious family menu, and even how to shop for the best, most healthful products. It truly is everything you need to know to get your family on the road to life-long good health.

Chapter 1
The Healthy Family

Healthy families are fortunate, but good health isn't just about luck. You have much more control over it than you may think. Attention to a healthy lifestyle is the first step. Nutrition and exercise are two elements that are easy to control, and they produce incredible results.

Nutrition and Happiness

Food is a part of our culture. It's important in our rituals, our religions, and our celebrations. We mark holidays, deaths, births, weddings, and milestones with food. We eat specific foods at specific times: popcorn at the movies, peanuts at the ball park, cake on our birthday. And in our darkest hours, we comfort ourselves with it. Our days revolve around food. We hold important meetings over lunch, rejuvenate ourselves over a coffee break, and relax with family over dinner. Food brings a lot of joy to our lives.

And food is necessary for life itself. Your body requires it. But just any old food won't do. The human body is very picky. For the body, food is not a source of joy but a source of fuel. All too often, people eat the wrong fuel, and that's harmful. Out of balance and lacking in substance, the human body deteriorates, both physically and mentally.

The goal is to get the right kind of fuel to keep yourself and your family running smoothly. A healthy diet meets all nutritional needs. It's not hard, but it does take forethought. Once you understand a few key elements, food can be both a source of joy and a source of energy.

Here it is in a nutshell: Eat plenty of fresh vegetables, fruits, and whole grains. These foods should make up the bulk of your diet. Choose lean meats and low-fat dairy foods, and avoid excess sugar. Last, but far from least, get plenty of exercise.

Benefits of a Healthy Diet

Eating well optimizes your body's ability to perform. It improves physical endurance as well as everyday tasks. Food affects your mental acuity, emotional outlook, personality, and overall sense of well-being. A healthy diet provides energy to function, as well as protection from chronic disease.

Specific Health Benefits

A healthy diet will minimize your risk of acquiring many of the chronic diseases currently plaguing our nation. Cardiovascular disease, stroke, diabetes, and certain cancers can all be connected in part to poor diets and failure to maintain healthy weight. Good nutrition improves the overall function of all aspects of the human body, from the way your blood flows to your ability to sleep.

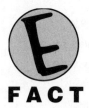

If an average overweight adult loses 10 percent of his weight, he can save as much as $5,000 in health care costs over a lifetime. Employers, too, are beginning to recognize the effects of obesity on health, and many are offering cash incentives to lose weight.

Personal Benefits

On a personal level, taking control of your health through diet is empowering. And if you are in control of your family's diet, the undertaking takes on even greater meaning. There is no better gift you can give your family than the gift of a healthy lifestyle. Developing healthy habits gives them an edge that will last a lifetime.

Healthy Variety

A nutritious diet does not have to be a boring diet. In fact, the healthiest diets are constantly evolving, trying and adding new foods with new combinations of nutrients. Once you have a clear understanding of what your body needs, you'll find a great deal of pleasure in experimentation and research.

Activity

A good diet is not enough. A healthy lifestyle also must include regular activity. You need activity to offset the calories you consume. Healthy foods give you the energy to be active, and in return, activity gives you an appetite for healthy food. When done properly, it is a beautiful symbiotic symphony of health.

Finding Your Sport

They only way to fit exercise into your life on a daily basis is to find something you enjoy. If you dread it, it can't help you. Joining a gym won't do you any good if you never go. You need to find what's right for you.

Finding exercise that fits your life has several components. It needs to fit regularly into your schedule. The skill you need to participate should be attainable, but not too easy. And whatever it is, it should present you with challenges and goals. There are dozens of activities out there that you can do alone or with friends. Don't limit your options to the equipment at the gym. Look around you. You'll find teams, clubs, parks, classes, and other people like you, looking for activity.

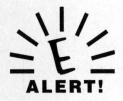

ALERT!

Beginning in adolescence, the amount of regular exercise girls get drops by more than 7 percent each year. Boys fare a little better, dropping only about 3 percent a year. You can thank the extra attention given to boys' sports for the disparity.

The Exercise Bonus

When you exercise on a regular basis, you quickly notice a boost in overall energy. This windfall is a powerful tool against stress. You sail through workdays more easily, with less fatigue and less tension. You'll find keeping up with small children less of a challenge, and you'll discover the drive to complete projects and consider new undertakings.

Your Ideal Weight

Our country as a whole is overweight. The American lifestyle has evolved into a sedentary pattern, with virtually no physical activity. Most Americans drive to work and sit at computers, then drive home and sit at the television. Kids get driven to school, where they sit all day, until they come home and sit at their desks or at their video games.

Meanwhile, technology improves, and the markets are packed with cheap, good-tasting, high-calorie foods. Coffee shops wait at every corner to help us with a boost of artificial energy and a cookie on the side. The fast food companies are conveniently located in our markets, shopping malls, and airports. They even supply our schools with lunches. It's no wonder two-thirds of Americans are overweight.

The technology of underdeveloped countries is not at our level, but neither is their rate of obesity. When people from these parts of the world immigrate to the West, their rate of weight gain quickly catches up to ours.

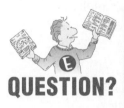

QUESTION?

How did people get so fat in the first place?
The human body was designed to enjoy and consume as much high-calorie food as possible. Humans are built to store extra calories until winter, or a time of famine, in pockets of fat. Unfortunately, human physiology has not compensated for technological advances.

Consequences of Being Overweight

Overweight people run higher risks for heart disease, high blood pressure, osteoporosis, osteoarthritis, infertility, stroke, diabetes, and numerous forms of cancer. Obesity is about to pass tobacco as the leading cause of preventable death. In 1998 Americans spent nearly $80 billion in obesity-related health care.

Regardless of how your weight compares to a table or chart, you know if you and your family need to pay more attention to nutrition. An ideal weight is one that you can maintain, that allows you to be active, provides energy throughout the day, and lets you sleep at night. What works for some does not necessarily work for all. You are an individual, and it's your unique lifestyle that determines your overall weight and health.

Where do you and your family fit in to this scenario? Are you active? Are you at a healthy weight? There are specific measurements you can make to determine exactly where you stand (see Chapter 21), but you probably have a pretty good idea already.

Battle of the Bulge

If you determine that you need to lose weight, there is only one way to do it. You must burn more calories than you consume. There are dozens of diet plans, programs, pills, and shakes vying for your dollar. But you can only lose the pounds by controlling portion sizes, understanding which foods your body needs, and incorporating exercise into your daily routine.

Cutting the calories takes attention, and burning them takes effort. There is no getting around it.

You can lose about a pound a week if you eliminate or burn 500 calories a day. To help you gauge this, an eight-ounce container of low-fat, plain yogurt has about 150 calories. People who run regularly burn about 100 calories per mile. Eat less, exercise more. Sounds simple enough, right?

Diet and Lifestyle

People's lifestyles vary, but for the most part, we are all busy. We work longer hours, our kids have more activities, and stay-at-home moms or dads are increasingly rare. Meals are home-cooked less frequently, and fast-food has become the norm. Finding nutritious meals and exercising more seems like just adding one more element to an already overloaded schedule. The secret is that by addressing your lifestyle in these areas, you will improve it.

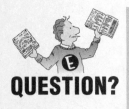

QUESTION?

How much do Americans spend in restaurants?
In the 1970s Americans spent about one-quarter of their food budgets eating out. In 1999 they were spending nearly half of what they make in restaurants. Imagine how much money could be saved by staying home even half the time!

Eat at Home

In order to maintain a nutritious lifestyle, the quality of the food consumed and its effect on the body must be the foremost concerns. Eating out is not only expensive, but in many cases it is the least healthy option. Cooking at home is the best way to ensure you and your family are eating right. But if you are already busy, cooking every meal may seem daunting. Planning can help. A weekly menu for meals and snacks will not only help you stay on track with a healthy diet, but it will also save you money. Save restaurants for special occasions.

Pay Attention to How You Eat

Make sure you and your family are eating for the right reasons. Overeating is easy to do in this day and age, but there are a few general rules you can follow to curb your munching habits.

- Don't eat while watching TV. When you're distracted, you lose track of how much you've eaten.
- Try not to eat and run. Take time to chew and enjoy the food you eat. You will feel more satisfied with less if you give your stomach time to recognize it is full.
- Eat the proper serving size. Even if you are famished, the proper serving size will satisfy you if you give it twenty minutes.
- Drink water when you're thirsty. Save sugary drinks like soda for special occasions. A single can of cola has around forty grams of sugar. Other styles of pop, like root beer or orange, have even more. Twelve grams of sugar is equal to about one tablespoon, so you are talking nearly four tablespoons, or a quarter cup per can!
- Keep only healthy snacks in the house. Snacks should be a part of your daily nutrition plan, curbing hunger until the next meal and providing a boost of energy. But the energy they give you should be long lasting. Energy from sugar and caffeine is not only fleeting, but it makes you feel worse when it's used up. Whole grains, vegetables, and fruits are better choices.

It's Never Too Late

The excuses for poor lifestyle choices are endless. "I don't have time" is the most common, but "I'm too old to change," or "I am stuck in my ways" are not far behind. Work, school, kids, and finances all vie for attention, and your health takes a back seat. But ironically, stress is alleviated as you begin eating healthfully and increasing activity.

Regardless of your age or your current condition, regular exercise and nutritious meals will increase your energy level. You will become more productive naturally, and you'll feel great.

Look at your current diet with objective eyes. Is it something you would share with your doctor? Your spouse? Your boss? Or do you think it needs improvement? If so, it's time to get serious about nutrition.

Understanding what foods you need to eat and why is the first step to overall health. It's not complicated. The following chapters break it down for you, step-by-step.

Once you have a grasp of the basics, you'll learn how to shop and cook for optimal nutrition. Even if you're not much of a cook now, you just might find the prospect of healthy cooking intriguing. Dozens of recipes and cooking tips are waiting to inspire you, along with some advice on getting and staying active.

Getting the Kids on Board

Teaching nutrition to kids is easy if you start from scratch, but not everyone has that luxury. Most parents tend to raise their kids as they were raised, and unfortunately everyone was not brought up by nutritionists. Interrupting the sugary soda and crunchy salty snack lives of older kids can be challenging.

When children are small and spending most of their time at home, it is easy to provide only natural, healthy foods. But the minute their care goes into the hands of someone else, be it day care, preschool, or Grandma, health-conscious parents need to go into double-overtime nutrition watch. Once refined sugars and flours are introduced to your child, the battle begins. Sweets are powerful things in the world of child care, and their use as reward has lifelong implications. To avoid this scenario, insist on maintaining control over your child's diet.

If you are already battling the junk food wars, there are ways to turn it around. They may take time, but they do work. Bringing kids into the process of planning, shopping, and cooking is an easy first step.

What's in It for Them?

Just like adults, kids like to see both sides and weigh the good and the bad. Even with young children, "because I said so" is not always effective. Results are better if they can see an upside to the changes you want them to make.

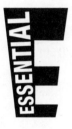

More than 60 percent of children eat too much fat. Less than 20 percent get enough vegetables. With an average of two trips to the drive-through each week, it's no wonder. Even so-called "healthy" fast food choices have hidden fat and sugar in dressings, breads, condiments, sodas, sides, and desserts.

Using outside influences is a great tactic. Find healthy role models for your children. Athletes are the obvious choices, but even TV and movie stars can work if they lead healthy lifestyles. Local coaches, dance instructors, and scout leaders also have healthy role model potential. Take a look at your child's activities and start pointing out the healthy active people in their lives.

Finally, give them incentive. It could be weight loss, increased strength for soccer, or better chances at cheerleading tryouts. Both kids and adults need incentive to do new, hard things. It may take some time, because unlike adults, a healthy future is not necessarily incentive enough. They do not necessarily see the potential for illness and disease. They are invincible in their own mind, so these goals are less effective. Help them find something tangible to work toward that is health or activity related. It may require finding them a new hobby or sport, but it's worth the effort. The payoff is a lifelong healthy lifestyle for your child.

Make Them Part of the Process

Give kids the power of knowledge. Explain the dietary guidelines, and use it to plan a menu together. Make a shopping list, and take them to the market. Teach them to read the labels and compare nutrients. (See Chapters 14, 15, 16, and 17 for more on kids and food.) Give them choices, within parameters, and make them responsible for monitoring their own diets. Most importantly, teach them how to cook. Even very young children can watch and help out in the kitchen and pick up important knowledge and skills.

From time to time you may need to let actions speak louder than words. A tummyache can be a powerful tool. Firsthand experience, including real physical results from poor choices, often work better than any incentive or role model. It will give you both a reference point from which to continue the work of daily nutrition. Even a sugar rush and crash can be useful if you are there to point out what is happening. Knowing the upside, and then downside, of unhealthy habits can be useful.

Most importantly, as a parent, you must never give in. Regardless of how much control you give them, you are still in charge. Don't slip into the fast and easy. It is your job to show them what a healthy lifestyle is. Being strict and vigilant in the early years will pay off with healthy active teens and adults.

Chapter 2
The Food Guide Pyramid

The United States Department of Agriculture (USDA) and the United States Department of Health and Human Services (HHS), and similar agencies worldwide, have addressed the nutritional needs of modern man and have provided handy guidelines to follow. Unfortunately, people don't. Every American over the age of seven recognizes the Food Guide Pyramid, but few can fill it in properly, and fewer still live by its guidelines. The perfect diet has been waiting patiently for you. It's time to pay attention!

The History of Government Guidelines

The Food Guide Pyramid has evolved over the years. Dietary guidelines were first instituted during World War II. In 1941, a national Food and Nutrition Board was convened to investigate the relationship between nutrition and national defense. The impact of nutrition on troops, prisoners, relief efforts, and the folks at home had never been fully investigated.

In the 1960s and 1970s kids were taught about square meals and the basic four food groups. The graphic for this curriculum was a square divided into four equal quadrants. Each space held one of the food groups: meat, bread, fruit and vegetables, and dairy.

This model had a few problems. First, there was little representation of the choices within each group. Therefore, chocolate milk, bacon, and white toast with grape jelly qualified as a well-rounded breakfast. The second problem was directly related to the graphic. Regardless of the servings suggested, the four squares suggested that each food group should be eaten in four equal proportions.

In 1980 the USDA revolutionized nutrition with the pyramid. This shape demonstrated, visually, the quantity of each food that should be consumed every day, and which foods should be limited.

The Pyramid Today

In 2005 the MyPyramid program was released, with even more detail, and had an added exercise component. The visual has changed, and there is an interactive website component, but the message is essentially the same. You need to eat more vegetables and grains, less fat and sugar. You should do this by consuming a variety of foods with good nutritional impact, while paying attention to quantity.

The MyPyramid website offers everyone a personal dietary plan. By simply inputting age, sex, weight, height, and level of physical activity, the site generates a complete listing of daily servings based on the number of calories each individual needs to maintain a healthy weight. Also available are meal-tracking worksheets, printable menus, and personal meal and activity assessments.

The downside of the MyPyramid plan is its need to appeal to the masses. Many foods, like milkshakes, refined grains, sugar, and oil are allowed, even though it is clear that these foods do not benefit overall health. Their inclusion does not adequately emphasize the need to replace refined foods with healthier options. People view words like *aim for* and *limit* as a green light to add junk food into their pyramid plan.

What to Eat and Why

Advice varies, and so do governmental recommendations. Each country has its preference, and many provide several guidelines based on specific diets, like the Mediterranean diet, or the vegan diet. Whichever you prefer, the main points are always the same; more grains and vegetables, less fat and sugar.

Grain and Cereal

The majority of your daily diet should consist of grains and cereals. This is the way your ancestors ate, and the way the world's healthiest cultures eat. Whole grains should take the largest space on your plate at every meal, every day.

Many dietary recommendations allow for some refined flours, but this is simply to make those diets more palatable. The healthiest diets aim for whole grains 100 percent of the time. Products made with refined white flour do not contribute enough fiber or nutrients. Our preference for white flour is one of the biggest contributors to our nation's health crisis.

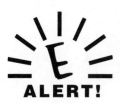
ALERT!

Only about one-quarter of Americans get their recommended vegetables. Thirty percent of the vegetables consumed by adults are potatoes. More than 20 percent of those potatoes are fried.

Vegetables and Fruits

Vegetables are the next crucial component of a healthy diet, and again, most Americans don't get enough. Adults should be eating a variety of brightly colored vegetables every day. The color is important, and should be varied, as each pigment carries different nutrients that you need. (Refer to the Vitamin Reference Chart in Chapter 4.) If all you eat is iceberg lettuce salad, you are missing crucial vitamins and minerals. Vegetables also provide fiber, a very valuable component of a healthy diet.

Fruit is important, but many people eat too much of it. Fruit contains vitamins and minerals, but many of the same nutrients are available in vegetables, and without the excess sugar. Between canned fruit, dried fruit, fruit fillings, and fruit juices, Americans overconsume fruit. All that sugar is an especially large contributor to childhood obesity. Fresh fruit should be consumed raw and whole. Other forms, especially juices, lose much of the nutritional benefit of their whole fruit counterparts.

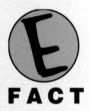

FACT

Americans consume about 200 pounds of meat every year. That works out to just over a half pound of meat a day. The recommended daily intake is five to six ounces. That means that annually people should eat over 60 pounds less than they do. Imagine the savings!

Protein

Protein is also overconsumed. Most Americans eat much more than their bodies need, and the most popular choices are the fattiest ones. This category includes meat, fish, poultry, eggs, beans, and nuts. A lighter diet, with less saturated fat, is the healthiest way to go. This means consuming lean meats like fish, and including more plant-based proteins on a regular basis.

Dairy

Dairy products are an important source of calcium for strong bones and teeth, but this food group is also loaded with saturated fat and milk sugar (lactose). Even if you find yourself eating a lot of dairy, you may not be getting enough calcium. Despite its appearance on the Food Guide Pyramid as an option, ice cream is not a good choice for calcium. The damage caused by the fat and sugar far outweigh any benefit from calcium. Remember, you can also find calcium in dark green vegetables like broccoli and collard greens, as well as fat-free dairy, soy products, and molasses. Choose dairy wisely, and be sure you are maximizing its benefit. Your body needs vitamin D to absorb calcium, which is only available from sunlight or through fortified supplements.

Junk Food

Much of the food people eat ends up in the junk food category, which is where they get into trouble. Fats and oils, refined sugars, and salt are the main culprits.

Fat and Oil

Fat insulates you, cushions your organs, and helps in the distribution of fat-soluble vitamins. But the typical American consumes far more fat than necessary. The naturally occurring fat in grains (such as wheat germ), fruits (olives and nuts), and animal products (fish, yogurt), is adequate for good health. Of course, that's only when these foods are eaten in the recommended amounts.

Sugar

Sugar, too, is essential for good nutrition. It gives you energy and helps your body function properly. But you were never meant to eat it in a refined state. Our bodies need the full benefit of the nutrients that come with a piece of fruit, or a bite of honey. These natural foods take time to digest, and are absorbed by the body slowly. When the nutrients are stripped away, the straight glucose goes right to work giving you instant energy. But that energy doesn't last long, and soon your body feels the resulting loss of energy in a "crash." The effect continues with unnatural cravings, unrelated to fueling the body.

Salt

Salt is a vital mineral, but your body needs less than a teaspoon a day, which is a fraction of what is consumed in a typical Western diet. Salt helps regulate body fluids and electrolytes, but too much can dehydrate you and is linked to high blood pressure and osteoporosis. You get an adequate amount of sodium naturally when you eat the recommended foods in the recommended quantities.

Serving Sizes

The amount of food you eat is just as important as the quality of the food you choose. A major contributor to our nation's overall poor health is lack of portion control. For years the serving size was buried in the small print, and often it is measured in quantities that you can't measure at home. Serving sizes vary with age but can be estimated easily by using everyday objects. The easiest measure is the palm of the hand. It is always with you, and it grows as you grow. This makes it easy to serve up the correct amount to both your toddler and your college linebacker.

Other objects you can use to estimate portion include:

- 1 slice of bread = 1 cassette tape
- ½ cup pasta or rice = a tennis ball
- 1 piece of fruit or cup of leafy greens = tennis ball
- ½ cup fruit or chopped vegetables = lightbulb
- 3 ounces lean meat = a deck of cards, or a checkbook
- 1 ounce cheese = 4 dice
- 2 tablespoons peanut butter = 1 ping pong ball

Number of Servings

Like the serving size, the number of servings varies from person to person. Adults need more than children, and active people need more than sedentary folks. The following list gives the range from five-year-old kids to adults. For younger children, please refer to Chapters 13 and 14.

Suggested Daily Servings

Food Group	Ages 5–10	Ages 11–15	Adult
Grain and Cereal	5–6 servings	6–7 servings	8–11 servings
Vegetables	4–5 servings	5–6 servings	6–8 servings
Fruits	2 servings	2–2½ servings	2½–3 servings
Dairy	2–2½ servings	2½ servings	3 servings
Meat/Protein	2 servings	2–2½ servings	3–4 servings

Grain and Cereal Servings

Aim for six to eight ounces of whole grains and cereals every day. An ounce of whole grains can be found in one slice of bread, one cup of cereal, or one-half cup of pasta or cooked grain such as rice or oats. Choose whole-grain cereals, whole-wheat pasta, whole-grain breads, brown rice, and straight whole grains like barley or quinoa.

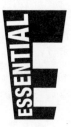

Quinoa (pronounced keen-wah) is an ancient grain from the Andes of South America. Together with corn and potatoes, it was a staple food of the Incas. Quinoa is one of the few plant foods that contain complete protein. (Read more about protein in Chapter 6.)

Vegetable Servings

Eat at least six servings of vegetables every day. Choose vegetables that are dark green and leafy, bright orange, red, and purple. Eat a variety of vegetables throughout the week, so your overall nutrient intake is broad. A serving includes one cup of leafy greens, one-half cup of chopped raw or cooked vegetables, or three-quarters of a cup of juice.

Fruit Servings

Limit fruit to two to three servings a day. While three-quarters of a cup of fruit juice counts as a serving, it is much healthier to eat a whole piece of fruit, which provides vital fiber. Eat the peels and skin of the fruit when possible, because much of the nutrients concentrate at the outer layer of the fruit. Dried fruits have concentrated nutrients, but also higher sugar levels, so beware. One serving of fruit is equivalent to one piece of fruit the size of a tennis ball, a quarter melon, a half grapefruit, or a quarter cup of dried fruit.

Dairy Servings

Keep daily dairy intake to two to three cups each day. Pick dairy with the lowest fat content. Milk, cheese, and plain yogurt are the best choices. Other dairy products, like flavored yogurts, chocolate milk, and ice cream, contain calcium, but also excessive fat and sugar. A serving is equivalent to one cup of milk or yogurt, a half cup of cottage cheese, or one and a half ounces of cheese.

ALERT!

Partially hydrogenated fat is artificially thickened vegetable oil. It contains trans fat, which is believed to not only increase bad cholesterol, but decrease good cholesterol. Trans fat is found in many foods, including margarine, salad dressings, cookies, and breads.

Protein Servings

Try to consume no more than four servings of lean protein every day. A serving of protein is found, approximately, in a half cup of cooked beans, one egg, two tablespoons of peanut butter, or a small chicken breast or hamburger at two and a half to three ounces. Beans and nuts are the healthiest choices. If you're a meat lover, look for lean meats, with skin and fat removed. Look for organic peanut butter with no added sugar.

Junk Servings

Fat and oil should be limited to no more than a half cup a day. Choose unsaturated oils, such as olive and peanut oils. Stay away from margarine and other partially hydrogenated oils.

Stay away from refined sugar as much as possible. Eat fresh and dried fruits for your sweet fix. Sweeten baked goods with honey, date sugar, or stevia—a sweetener extracted from an herb (called stevia, sweetleaf, or sugarleaf) that is 300 times sweeter than granulated sugar.

Water

You've been told all your life: Drink lots of water! Dehydration causes fatigue, lack of concentration, mood swings, dry mouth, lightheadedness, and eventually loss of consciousness, so keeping well hydrated is a good idea. The best advice is to drink water with meals, and occasionally throughout the day, to maintain good fluid balance and to stay mentally alert. Beverages with sugar; caffeine; or artificial flavors, colors, and preservatives do not rehydrate you, and will generally dehydrate you.

The Exercise Component

Today's Food Guide Pyramid takes exercise seriously—so much so that a little stairclimbing figure is highlighted in the graphic. The recommended amount of exercise varies by age, but most recommendations hover around thirty minutes per day. Unfortunately, this number is misleading.

A healthy active person should warm up for ten minutes, work out for thirty minutes at their target heart rate (see Chapter 20), and then cool down for ten minutes. If you are trying to lose weight, the time at target heart rate is increased. Kids require at least an hour of daily exercise.

It is difficult for some people to figure out how to add exercise to already busy daily routines. The only real way to do it is to make it enjoyable. You've got to want to do it. There are several ways to go about this.

Try It All

You may not be exercising now because you haven't found the activity that lights your fire. There are so many options available you're bound to find one that suites you. There are the standard options, like running, biking, and swimming, but there are also lots of sports, like racquetball, tennis, soccer, football, rugby, hockey, ice skating, skate- and snowboarding, surfing, rock climbing, and even dodgeball. Join a league, or start your own and challenge coworkers to a lunchtime scrimmage.

Friends

If you're a social person, exercise is a great way to meet and get to know people. There are health clubs and gyms all over the place, ready to sign you up with lots of attractive and interesting members. The local YMCA has lower fees than many premium gyms, and typically offers all sorts of classes in addition to the standard equipment.

That being said, exercise does not have to cost you money. Getting out and walking or running every day is free (until you decide you need better shoes). Organize a bike ride with some buddies, or take your dog for a hike.

Going Solo

If you'd rather keep to yourself, you can still go walking or running. Get your favorite upbeat music on an MP3, portable disc, iPod, or even a radio headset. Or go to the library and check out a yoga or belly dancing tape. Then you can shake it in the privacy of your own room.

Besides finding an activity you like, you'll need some motivation, especially when you are just starting. Friends can be helpful, but it's easy to talk someone into being lazy, too. A better motivator is an event or situation. A high school or family reunion, holiday party, wedding, new job, new town, or new school can be powerful motivation to work toward a new you. And of course, there is always romance. Looking for a new relationship, or revving up an old one, can really get your juices pumping and motivation sparking.

Chapter 3
Food Labels

Once you start caring about the food you eat, you will find that reading labels is irresistible. Everything you need to know about the nutritional components of the food you are buying is conveniently located in one spot. You can compare and contrast to your heart's content. This chapter will tell you how to interpret the information you find on food labels and what to look for and avoid when you go grocery shopping.

Food Label History

Food labels have been mandatory in the United States since the 1990s, but they have been in the making since the 1860s. What began as an agricultural research and development project quickly morphed into a food safety organization. After the Civil War, as interstate commerce picked up, there was a need for standardized weights, measures, and manufacturing practices.

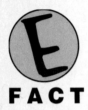

FACT

After the Civil War, each state had its own food regulations. It was common for food companies to produce different versions of the same product, in varying degrees of quality, to comply with different state laws.

By the 1870s concern for quality of traded goods prompted the pure food movement. These activists urged lawmakers to make food adulteration a crime. At the time, chemical preservatives went uncontrolled, milk was unpasteurized, and ice was the only form of refrigeration. Cottonseed oil was routinely sold as lard, and glucose syrup made from wheat and corn was used as a cheaper form of sugar. And unbeknownst to the consumer, medical "tonics" routinely contained opium, morphine, cocaine, and heroin. In 1903, volunteer "poison squads" ate foods tainted with chemical preservatives to demonstrate their effect on human health.

The Jungle

Frequent food-related illness and death fueled the pure food movement with the help of women's groups and magazines, which frequently printed articles reporting on the horrors of food contamination.

Finally, in 1906, a novel entitled *The Jungle*, by Upton Sinclair, described the horrific conditions of the Chicago meatpacking industry. That same year, the Pure Food and Drug Act and the Meat Inspection Act were passed, and a federal agency was created to protect consumers. The Bureau of Chemistry enforced the law, but in order to allow them more resources for agricultural research, the enforcement shifted to a new agency, the Federal Drug and Insecticide Agency. The department was so-named until the 1930s, when insecticide control was diverted, and it became the FDA.

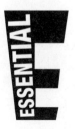

Curiously, *The Jungle* began as a social commentary on the labor movement in the United States. While the majority of the book's content revolved around appalling work conditions and unfair labor practices, it was the treatment of the meat itself that garnered the most attention, much to Mr. Sinclair's disappointment.

Modern FDA

Regulation of packaged food began in 1913 with legislation requiring that foods have clearly labeled weight, measure, or numerical count of their contents. In the 1930s, generalized quality ratings were required. They weren't very telling, as the only requirement was either "standard," "below standard," or "above standard." Not until the 1960s were nutritional content and an ingredients list required on packages. The FDA reviewed every label for accuracy.

In 1990 the Nutritional Label Education Act regulated health claims made on food labels, such as "light" and "low-fat." In 1992 the Nutrition Facts Panel first appeared, showing per-serving nutritional information.

How to Read Nutrition Labels

There are several key areas of a food label to look at. The first and most obvious is the front of the package. There you will find graphics designed to appeal to a specific consumer. For instance, bright colors and cute or goofy characters are aimed at kids. Also on the front are the product's claims: "Tastes Great" and " New and Improved" are the tame ones. It's the health claims that consumers need to pay attention to. "Heart-Healthy," "Whole Grain," and "Less Sugar" are claims designed to draw the attention of health conscious, but not necessarily nutritionally savvy, shoppers.

Also on the package somewhere will be a list of ingredients, and the nutrition facts panel. It is these last two elements that consumers should be paying attention to.

The Nutrition Facts Panel

Nutrients on the facts panel were chosen by their importance in relation to modern health issues. New listings appear as health concerns change. For example, the listing for trans fat is a relatively recent addition. Placement on the label is an indication of importance, too. For instance, sodium is not listed with the other minerals and micronutrients, but up high, next to cholesterol, because many people need to monitor their sodium intake.

The labels are placed on every food package, either vertically or horizontally. Sometimes you have to search a bit, as folds in the packaging can hide it. Sometimes, too, the label is on a box, but not on individually packaged contents.

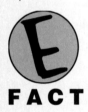

FACT

Most food served for immediate consumption, such as that sold in bakeries or delis, or served on airplanes or in hospitals, is not required to be labeled. But if a restaurant makes specific health and nutrient claims, then labels (typically on a separate sheet) must be provided upon request.

Serving Size

The top of the panel lists the serving information. The serving size is the quantity of product that the facts are based on. The facts are not based on the entire package. If you do not read the serving size, the rest of the information is useless.

Serving sizes are often shocking. For instance, a regular four-inch bagel may constitute over two servings, while a serving of cookies may be just one cookie. Do not be misled by a low calorie count. Check the serving size before you get excited.

Don't forget to take the food's preparation, if any, into consideration. Serving size may be before or after water or other ingredients are added. This information will also be printed clearly in the serving size area of the label.

Servings per Container

This little bit of information is useful if you tend to eat an entire package of food in one sitting. It will tell you how many servings are contained in the package. All it takes is some easy math to figure out just how many servings, and thus how many calories and grams of fat, were in that bag of chips you just wolfed down.

Percent Daily Value

Daily values, (also known as daily reference values, or DRVs) show you how much of the daily recommended nutrients are in the product. The figure is given as a percent of a designated amount of nutrients required for a 2,000-calorie-per-day diet. The recommendations are high and considered the most that would be healthful for adults.

The percentage listed on the label is based on a recommendation of total daily nutrients. These daily nutrient percentages are as follows:

- Fat should constitute 30 percent of calories
- Saturated fat should constitute 10 percent of calories
- Carbohydrates should constitute 60 percent of calories
- Protein should constitute 10 percent of calories
- Fiber is based on 13 grams daily

If you are on a special diet, these percentages will not apply. (See Chapter 19 for more information on special diets.)

RDI

The term *recommended daily allowance* is being replaced by *reference daily intake* (RDI). Recommended daily allowance was prompted by investigations into diet and nutrition during World War II. Information gained in those studies was put to use in the armed forces, the civilian population, and in overseas relief efforts. The RDIs are the equivalent to the RDAs, and are used to determine the daily reference value percentages.

Calories

Calories measure energy. They are determined by burning a weighed portion of food, and measuring the heat it produces. Different nutrients contain different calories. Carbohydrates and protein each contain four calories per gram, fat has nine calories per gram, and alcohol has seven calories per gram.

In prepared foods with numerous ingredients and varying portion size, the calorie designation is useful and welcome information. However, be careful not to limit your label reading to the calorie section. Low calories often mean low nutrition. Knowledge of calories is only a small part of your healthy eating arsenal.

Fat, Carbohydrates, and Protein

A general listing for fat is given, followed by sublistings for saturated fat and trans fat, two forms of fatty acids that should be as close to zero as possible in healthy diets. (See Chapter 8 for more information about fat.) There are also listings for cholesterol and sodium, two nutrients that should be limited as well.

Carbohydrates are listed as a total figure, as well as being separated into fiber and sugar. Fiber is a carbohydrate that, while indigestible, is still vital for good health. Fiber helps keep digestion flowing, and maintains normal cholesterol and blood sugar levels. There is no daily value percentage for sugar, because it is not a recommended nutrient.

Protein is generally not a nutrient Americans need to be concerned with. We get plenty of it, so listing its daily value percentage is not required unless the product is marketed as a high-protein food, as in baby food or meal replacements. Often the grams per serving is all that is listed.

Vitamins and Minerals

The only required listings in this section are vitamin A, vitamin C, calcium, and iron. These micronutrients are often deficient in the average diet. Products may choose to add more information on vitamins and minerals if the product contains significant quantities.

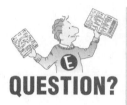

QUESTION?

What are micro- and macronutrients?
Vitamins and minerals are considered micronutrients because only small quantities are necessary for good health. (Micro is from the Greek *mikros*, meaning "small.") Carbohydrates, protein, fat, and water are considered macronutrients, as you require a much larger quantity. (Macro is from the Greek *makros*, meaning "long.")

Recommended Daily Limits

On larger packages, just below the vitamins and minerals you may find a list of the daily limits of nutrients. These numbers, listed as quantities in grams, are based on a 2,000- and 2,500-calorie diet. This is a nice reminder of overall dietary needs. For a 2,000-calorie diet, the daily limits are as follows:

- Total fat should not exceed 65 grams
- Total saturated fat should not exceed 20 grams
- Total cholesterol should not exceed 300 milligrams
- Total sodium should not exceed 2,400 milligrams

Nutritional Claims

It's hard to find a label that doesn't make some sort of claim hoping to make it into your shopping cart. But when you see the words "free" or "light" on the label, can you believe them? According to the FDA, you can. Manufacturers are required to provide scientific evidence before they are allowed to make claims on labels. There are twelve words that are strictly regulated: free, low, reduced, less, lean, extra lean, light/lite, more, fewer, high, good source, and healthy.

Free

A label claiming to be calorie free must contain less than five calories per serving. Sodium-free, sugar-free, and fat-free foods must contain less than .5 grams per serving. "Cholesterol free" means the product has less than 2 milligrams of cholesterol per serving, and 2 grams or less saturated fat per serving.

Low

"Low calorie" means the product has forty calories or less per serving. "Low fat" products must have 3 grams of fat or less per serving. "Low-cholesterol" means less than 20 milligrams per serving and 2 grams or less of saturated fat per serving. "Low sodium" must have 140 milligrams or less per serving. "Very low sodium" means 35 milligrams or less.

Reduced

A product labeled "reduced" must have at least 25 percent less of the nutrient than the food it is referencing. For example, reduced-fat salad dressing must have 25 percent less fat than regular salad dressing. The synonym is "fewer."

Less

A product labeled "less" must have 25 percent less of a nutrient than the food it is referencing. For example, chicken broth labeled as having less sodium must have 25 percent less sodium than regular chicken broth.

Lean and Extra-Lean

"Lean" foods must have 10 grams or less of total fat, 4.5 grams or less of saturated fat, and 95 milligrams or less of cholesterol per serving or per 100 grams. "Extra-lean" foods can have no more than 5 grams total fat, 2 grams saturated fat, and 95 milligrams cholesterol.

Light or Lite

Products labeled "light" must have one-third fewer calories per serving than the food it is referencing, or 50 percent less fat than the reference food. If the product gets over 50 percent of its calories from fat, it must reduce the fat by another 50 percent to carry the "light" descriptor. Light sodium means the product has 50 percent less sodium per serving.

More

Products labeled "more" must contain at least 10 percent of the daily reference value of the nutrient in question. Synonyms include "fortified," "enriched," "added," "extra," and "plus."

Fewer

Claims of "fewer" are the same as those for reduced. The product must contain at least 25 percent less of the nutrient than the referenced product.

High

Products with "high" on the label must contain 20 percent of the daily reference value or more of vitamins, minerals, fiber, or protein.

Good Source

If a product claims to be a "good source" of something, it must have 10–19 percent of the daily value of that vitamin, mineral, fiber, or protein.

Healthy

Perhaps the most crucial word of all, the "healthy" claim, has several criteria. It must provide at least 10 percent of the daily value of vitamins, minerals, fiber, or protein. If it is a meal product (meant to serve as an entire meal, such as a frozen dinner), it must contain 10 percent of the daily value of at least two of those nutrients. Sodium may not exceed 360 milligrams, or 480 milligrams for a meal product. The product must also follow the criteria for low–fat, low–saturated fat, and low cholesterol.

Health Claims

Claims regarding specific health issues are strictly regulated by the FDA. The words "may" and "might" must appear as a part of such claims.

These claims are powerful. If a product meets the criteria, its label can state that the product may prevent cancer, or brain damage, or heart disease. These claims are exciting, but it's important to note that these products do nothing in terms of prevention unless combined with a healthy lifestyle.

Many products link themselves to prevention of a certain disease. Claims regarding osteoporosis must contain 200 milligrams, or 20 percent of the daily value of calcium, and must be low in fat. Low-fat, low–saturated fat, and low-cholesterol foods and extra-lean meats may claim to help prevent cancer and coronary heart disease. These claims can also be made for high-fiber foods that meet the "low-fat" criterion and the "good source" criterion for fiber and vitamin A or vitamin C. Soy protein products for the prevention of cancer must meet the low-fat criterion and carry at least 6.25 grams of soy protein per serving.

Other Claims

"Percent fat-free" products must meet the low-fat or fat-free criterion. The percentage used must reflect the amount of fat in 100 grams of the product.

Some products try to imply health. Stating a product is made with a nutritious product, such as soy or bran, is not allowed unless the product can meet the "good source" criterion.

The term "fresh" can be used if the product is raw or unprocessed. This means it has never been frozen or heated, and it contains no preservatives. This is used in products like fresh mozzarella cheese, sold in brine, and dated for freshness. Fresh-frozen products are frozen while still fresh in the orchards or on fishing boats. Some blanched and low-irradiated products may be called fresh as well.

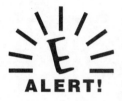

ALERT!

Claims that imply health through inclusion of certain ingredients are particularly problematic when new health and nutrition reports are in the news. To be sure what you're buying is all that it claims, check the FDA website, *www.fda.gov*, for up-to-the-minute information.

The Ingredients List

Ingredients are listed on products by weight, from most to least. The food's main ingredient will be listed first. This is important to know, especially when looking at sweetened foods. If the food contains only one ingredient, such as a bag of dried beans, no ingredient list is required.

Ingredient lists are vital to people with allergies. It is estimated that 8 percent of children in the United States have food allergies. Of these, 90 percent are caused by one of eight foods: milk, eggs, peanuts, wheat, soy, fish, shellfish, and tree nuts. These eight foods must be listed on an ingredients list if they are used in the product. Color additives, too, must be acknowledged in the ingredients list by name, as well as soy-based flavor enhancers and milk derivatives called caseinates, commonly used in nondairy products. Beverages that claim to contain a specific juice must list the percentage of that juice.

Familiarizing yourself with the ingredients list, the food facts panel, and the labeling laws is an eye-opening experience. Take a look at the foods you have in your cupboard right now and see how they rate. You may be surprised.

Chapter 4
All about Vitamins

Vitamins are called micronutrients because they are required in small amounts. But the contribution they make to your overall health is gigantic. Vitamins are found in small amounts in the foods you eat, and some are created in your body. And because they are so varied, you must consume a variety of foods to maintain balanced nutrition. In this chapter, you'll learn all you need to know about the different vitamins and how much you need of each.

The Importance of Daily Vitamin Intake

Vitamins are a necessary component of a healthy diet. They are considered essential nutrients because our bodies either do not make them, or do not make enough of them. They are essential for normal body functions like cell growth, blood cell production, hormone and enzyme synthesis, energy metabolism, and proper functioning of body systems, including the immune system, nervous system, circulatory system, and reproductive system.

Since no single food contains all the vitamins you need, you must obtain them through a variety of foods. You can take a pill that contains vitamins, but it is always preferable to get them the natural way. The reason is twofold. If you take a supplement because you assume your diet is poor, you may not be supplementing the right nutrients. More importantly, getting your vitamins by eating healthy foods provides the body with many other nutrients necessary for good health, including fiber, carbohydrates, protein, and water.

Fat-Soluble Vitamins

Four of the essential vitamins are fat soluble. That means that they dissolve in fat, not water, and are stored in fatty tissue and in the liver. Because they can be stored for long periods of time, people consuming a well-balanced diet do not need to supplement them. In fact, because these vitamins hang around, they are more prone to toxicity than the water-soluble vitamins.

A normal amount of fat in the diet is necessary to metabolize these fat-soluble vitamins. They are absorbed through the large intestine, and there must be some fat present for successful absorption. After absorption, these vitamins are stored in the liver until needed.

Vitamin A

Also known as retinol, vitamin A is primarily found in animal foods, including dairy products, fish, liver, and egg yolks. It has a pro-vitamin, called beta carotene, which is found in vegetables with orange pigment, like carrots, sweet potatoes, and apricots, as well as some dark, leafy greens including spinach and kale.

As you may have guessed by its pseudonym, beta carotene, and its presence in carrots, vitamin A is important for the health of your eyes. It is vital for night vision and the adjustments the eye regularly makes to various light levels. Vitamin A also helps keep skin healthy, promotes healthy bone and tooth growth, and is vital for proper cell division and reproduction. It also strengthens and moistens mucous membranes, which helps resist infections.

Deficiencies are rare, but symptoms may include night blindness and seriously dry and itchy skin, as well as slow tooth and bone growth.

Signs of vitamin A toxicity include dry itchy skin, nausea, and headache. Excessive beta carotene has been known to turn skin a pale orange.

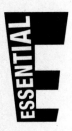

A pro-vitamin is not a vitamin that has renounced its amateur status. Also known as a vitamin precursor, pro-vitamins are organic compounds that, once ingested, the body converts into a vitamin.

Vitamin D

Because it is naturally synthesized by sunlight on your skin, vitamin D is sometimes called the sunshine vitamin. Ten minutes in the sun is enough to give you your daily dose. During the Industrial Revolution, when people began spending more time indoors, and the skies were clouded by pollutants, rickets was rampant. Rickets is a disease in which bones do not harden properly and become soft and painful. Scientists suspected a dietary deficiency along the same lines as scurvy, and it was soon found that cod liver oil eliminated the disease. It was also noted that long doses of sunshine were restorative.

Vitamin D's main function is to control the absorption of calcium, which promotes the hardening of bones and teeth. Deficiency in vitamin D leads to rickets in children, and a similar affliction in adults, osteomalacia. It might also be a contributor to osteoporosis. These conditions occur when bone mineralization is impaired, keeping bones from hardening properly. As a result, they become soft, weak, painful, and fragile. People living with minimal sunshine, in areas with lots of cloud or fog cover, spending much of their time indoors, or covered with sunblock, are likely candidates for vitamin D deficiency. Because of this, vitamin D has been added to many products, most notably milk. Small amounts occur naturally in a few foods, including sardines, herring, and cod liver oil.

Toxicity of vitamin D in mild forms leads to nausea, irritability, and weight loss. Severe cases result in mental and physical growth retardation, calcium in the blood, and kidney damage.

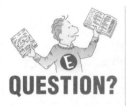

QUESTION?

Will sunblock prevent vitamin D absorption?
Proper use of sunblock, with a sun protection factor (SPF) of 15, will deflect or absorb all but 7 percent of the UVB rays that synthesize vitamin D (and cause skin cancer). But most people fail to apply sunblock properly. You need at least an ounce, or about two tablespoons, and it should be applied fifteen to twenty minutes before going outdoors so that it has ample time to penetrate. Most people apply it too late, and too sparingly, cutting its effectiveness in half. Chances are you're still getting your vitamin D.

Vitamin E

This vitamin is a powerful antioxidant. Additionally it works to protect vitamins A and C and red and white blood cells, promotes iron metabolism, and helps maintain nervous system tissue. Some past studies suggest that vitamin E can slow the development of heart disease, but current wisdom notes that diets high in all antioxidants lower risks of cancer and disease. You'll find vitamin E in seeds, whole grains, and nuts.

Deficiency in vitamin E is rare, but toxicity can occur. Symptoms include nausea and gastrointestinal disorders.

Vitamin K

This vitamin is sometimes called the band-aid vitamin because its primary function is in the clotting of blood. In fact, the K comes from the Danish word *koagulation*. Vitamin K also helps hold calcium in your bones. It is naturally produced by bacteria in the intestines, but it can also be found in dark, leafy green vegetables, like turnip greens, spinach, broccoli, and cabbage.

Deficiency results in excessive bleeding. Because vitamin K is formed by bacteria in the intestines, bacteria-killing antibiotics can be problematic. Also, because it is fat soluble, people that have difficulties digesting fat may become deficient.

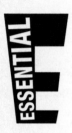

Antioxidants can slow, prevent, and reverse damage done by oxidation. Oxidation is an electron transfer process (the loss of electrons by a molecule, atom, or ion), which can produce free radicals. Free radicals damage body cells and tissues.

Water-Soluble Vitamins

Water-soluble vitamins dissolve in water, and, because your body is made mostly of water, they cannot be stored. Once ingested, they are easily lost through sweat and urine. In food they are easily lost by poor storage and excessive cooking. Therefore, you need a continuous supply of these vitamins to stay healthy.

Institutional food is a frequent source of water-soluble vitamin deficiency. Cooking in such quantities frequently results in overcooked and reheated foods, which causes considerable loss of these nutrients.

Eight of the water-soluble vitamins were once thought to be the same compound, designated by early scientists as vitamin B. Later, it was shown to be several compounds, and broken up into a group commonly known as the B complex. Cooking vegetables in water is the best way to eliminate water-soluble vitamins. Unless you are making soup, and therefore plan to consume the cooking liquid, you should steam or quickly sauté your veggies over high heat. Canned vegetables, which are subjected to high heat in the canning process, are short on vitamins, too.

B_1—Thiamin

The main function of thiamin is its role in creating an enzyme (thiamin pyrophosphate) that is essential in the conversion of food to energy. It also contributes to the proper functioning of the nervous system by keeping the heart muscle elastic. Thiamin is found in whole grains, seeds, legumes, pork, and liver, and is fortified in many food products.

B_2—Riboflavin

This vitamin's most important job is cell respiration. Oxygen and food molecules enter a cell, and there, enzymes release the food's and oxygen's energy. These enzymes contain riboflavin. If riboflavin is absent, the cells cannot release enough energy.

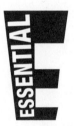

Serious athletes, who are regularly expending a lot of energy, may benefit from increased riboflavin, due to its role in protein synthesis and energy metabolism.

Riboflavin also regulates cell growth, helps in the production of red blood cells, and is important for healthy hair and skin. It helps the immune system by making antibodies and keeping mucous membranes healthy and able to fight off germs. Some studies suggest that it can be useful in reducing migraine headaches.

Riboflavin is found in dark green vegetables and whole grains. It is also found in milk products, especially cottage cheese and yogurt. This is because riboflavin is easily destroyed by light, and packages of cottage cheese and yogurt are typically opaque.

Deficiency results in dry cracked skin, especially around the mouth and nose. Eyes can also become sensitive to light. There is no known toxicity.

B₃—Niacin

Here is another enzyme-producing B vitamin that is used in the release of energy from cells. In addition, niacin helps control glucose levels in blood, and it is necessary for healthy nervous and digestive systems.

Niacin is found in high-protein foods such as fish, meat, poultry, peanuts, and in whole grains. When corn became a staple food of the poor throughout Europe, South America, and the southern United States, the niacin-deficiency disease pellagra became widespread. Symptoms include dermatitis, skin lesions, swollen tongue, mental confusion, aggression, and dementia.

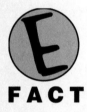

FACT

Hominy, which is corn soaked in lye (lye is an alkali solution traditionally derived from ash), is the basis for corn tortillas, posole, and grits. The alkali makes the tryptophan in corn available as a nutrient, and corrects corn's niacin deficiency.

The best source of niacin is from the amino acid tryptophan, found in much of the animal protein you eat. Half of this amino acid is converted to niacin in the body. Vegans, who do not eat animal protein, run the risk of niacin deficiency.

B₅—Pantothenic Acid

This vitamin, found in every food and made by intestinal bacteria, is important in the creation of enzymes that enable the conversion of fat and carbohydrates into energy. It is also part of hormone and red blood cell formation.

There is no recommended amount because it is so readily available in food. The best source for B₅ is organ meat, but it is also plentiful in salmon, whole grains, eggs, beans, and milk. Be aware that frozen meat that has been defrosted loses half of its pantothenic acid.

Deficiency has only been witnessed in lab studies, and results in fatigue, mood swings, nausea, and cramps.

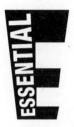

Some endurance athletes claim pantothenic acid helps them train harder. Extra B_5 is taken to better release energy from fats and carbs and incur less lactic acid buildup. To date there has not been extensive research into these claims, however.

B_6—Pyridoxine

This vitamin builds over sixty enzymes, working for your immune and nervous systems and helping form red blood cells. It turns the protein you eat into proteins your body needs and helps convert carbohydrates into energy.

B_6 is best found in high-quality protein foods like chicken and fish. It occurs in dairy, but not as much, so again, vegetarians are frequently deficient. Deficiency symptoms include getting sick frequently because the immune system is weakened. Also common with B_6 deficiency is anemia, a low red blood cell count.

Some medications cause excretion of B_6, including drugs for high blood pressure, asthma, arthritis, and birth control, as does alcohol. Toxicity is possible with large doses, more than 2,000 milligrams per day. B_6 toxicity causes neurological damage. Symptoms can include tingling or numbness, and difficulty walking.

B_9—Folic Acid

This vitamin is essential for strong bodies. It aids in protein metabolism, helps new red blood cell formation, and has been shown to prevent spine and brain birth defects and lower the risk of heart disease.

Beans are a good source of folic acid, as is spinach, asparagus, and chicken or beef liver. As with all water-soluble vitamins, nutrients are easily lost in cooking. Deficiencies cause anemia, nausea, sore tongue, headache, and weakness. Because B vitamins work together, being low in one usually means you are low in them all.

Deficiency in folic acid can also be a sign of cancer. Cancer cells use up folic acid to fuel their cell division. Toxicity from folic acid is not a concern, as excess is excreted. Too much folic acid, however, can mask a rare type of anemia caused by a deficiency of B_{12}.

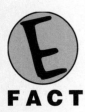

FACT

Anemia is the most common blood disorder, classified as a deficiency of red blood cells or hemoglobin. It can be caused by loss of blood, destruction of red blood cells, or insufficient red blood cells. Symptoms include weakness, fatigue, lack of concentration, and in extreme cases, shortness of breath and heart failure.

B_{12}—Colabamin

Found only in animal foods, B_{12} is crucial to maintaining healthy red blood cells, immune systems, and the development of genetic material. It helps the nervous system by strengthening the fatty layer of nerve cells.

Your body absorbs only about half of the B_{12} you take in, so intake is double what you need. Because it is found in animal foods, vegetarians may need supplements, as may the elderly. As people age, their bodies have difficulty absorbing B_{12}, and the difficulty increases the older you get. Additionally, potassium supplements interfere with B_{12} absorption.

A condition known as pernicious anemia is caused by B_{12} deficiency. Other deficiency symptoms include pins and needles in hands and feet, numbness, depression, memory loss, and dementia.

Biotin, Choline, and Inositol

These are vitamins that you do not need to consume because they are made in adequate amounts by bacteria in your intestines. Toxicity is unknown and deficiency is rare, but they are worth mentioning, as they work closely with the other B vitamins, converting your food into energy. Biotin in particular helps you utilize fats and proteins. Choline and inositol work together in the formation of neurotransmitters, crucial for brain function, cell membranes, and to move fats out of your liver.

Vitamin C

This is arguably the king of all vitamins. Also known as ascorbic acid, vitamin C plays an important role for over 300 functions in the body. It is the body's main antioxidant, it protects the immune system, helps build collagen for connective tissues, and heals wounds. Vitamin C is vital in the absorption of iron and calcium. It helps maintain blood vessels, bones, teeth, and the formation of brain hormones.

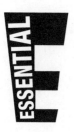

Rose hips are a potent source of vitamin C. Classically used for jellies and teas, rose hips are the fruit of the rose plant. They appear as red, orange, or purple balls, left on the bush after the flower has died. Remove the seeds and skin and dry or puree the inner pulp. Rose hip tea is available at health food stores.

Vitamin C is associated with citrus fruit, which carries a lot of it, but it is also found in leafy greens, especially watercress, kiwi fruit, peppers, potatoes, broccoli, strawberries, and tomatoes. Vitamin C requirements are increased by smoking, stress, allergies, birth control pills, antibiotics, and fever.

Deficiency results in scurvy, a disease whose symptoms include spots on legs, sore and bleeding gums, tooth loss, wounds that reopen, and eventually death. British sailors were given a daily ration of lime to prevent scurvy (that's where the nickname "limey" originated). Because such deficiencies are easily treatable with vitamin C, fatalities are rare.

Vitamin and Nutrient Quantities

If ingested in large quantities, all nutrients can be dangerous. Safe intake levels vary, and as such, the dietary reference intake (DRI) is the best current assessment of safe quantities. Many people are of the opinion that if something is good for you, a larger quantity is even better. In an attempt to deter people from this misconception, and prevent the possibility of side effects, DRI is available for all vitamins and minerals.

Following is an easy-to-use list of the vitamins, their functions, sources, and the recommended daily intakes. The measurements are listed in various forms because there is not one standard unit, especially for such small amounts. A milligram (mg) is a unit you are probably familiar with. It is 1/1,000 of a gram. Micrograms (mcg) are more unusual. A microgram is equivalent to 1/1,000,000 of a gram. Pretty small indeed.

An international unit (IU) is a bit more complicated. Used to measure drugs and vitamins, the IU of a substance varies with the biological activity and potency of the substance. The IU to mg conversion rate differs with each substance, but each substance ratio is set, having been determined by the World Health Organization. For example, 1 IU of vitamin A is equal to .03 mcg of retinol, and 0.6 mcg of beta carotene. 1 IU of vitamin C is equal to 50 mcg of ascorbic acid.

This simple conversion can help you better understand the amounts referred to in the following table: 1 gram is equal to .035 ounce. One ounce is equal to 28.35 grams.

Vitamin Reference Chart

Vitamin	RDI	Major Functions	Best Food Sources
Vitamin A	5,000 IU	maintains healthy eyes, skin, bones, and teeth	orange vegetables, fruits, and green leafy vegetables
Vitamin D	400 IU	calcium absorption	small oily fish, cod liver oil, fortified milk

Vitamin	RDI	Major Functions	Best Food Sources
Vitamin E	30 IU	antioxidant, protects red blood cells	seeds, whole grains, nuts
Vitamin K	70 mcg	blood clotting	green leafy vegetables
Vitamin C	60 mg	antioxidant, iron absorption, formation of collagen, bones, teeth, red blood cell formation	citrus fruit, tomatoes, bell peppers, kiwi, papaya
B_1—Thiamin	1.5 mg	energy production	whole grains, seeds, nuts
B_2—Riboflavin	1.7 mg	energy production, healthy eyes and skin	dark green vegetables, whole grains, cottage cheese, yogurt
B_3—Niacin	20 mg	energy production, proper functioning of central nervous system	meat, fish, poultry, whole grains, peanuts
B_5—Pantothenic Acid	10 mg	energy production, amino acid metabolism, proper adrenal gland function, synthesis of neurotransmitters	organ meats, salmon, eggs
B_6—Pyridoxine	2 mg	energy production, fat metabolism, red blood cell and hemoglobin synthesis	meat, fish, poultry, milk
B_7—Biotin	300 mcg	energy production, amino acid metabolism	liver, egg yolks, brewer's yeast, nuts, whole grains
B_9—Folic Acid	400 mcg	red blood cell formation, metabolism of fat, amino acids, DNA and RNA synthesis	beans, spinach, liver
B_{12}—Cobalamin	6 mcg	proper functioning of central nervous system, DNA synthesis	meat, fish, poultry, eggs, milk

Supplements

Nearly half of all Americans take dietary supplements, but less that 10 percent take them under a doctor's care. This multibillion-dollar industry makes its money from claims, legitimate or not, of increased performance, weight loss, resistance to illness, stamina, and improved mood. But it all boils down to adequate nutrient intake.

The very best way to get your nutrients is to eat them in a variety of foods. Science is always learning, and while we understand much about nutrients in food, there are certainly elements in food that are not yet understood. This is especially true in the study of trace minerals.

Sometimes supplements are necessary. Women who are pregnant, nursing, or premenopausal can benefit from vitamin supplements. People on special diets, such as vegetarians, or those consuming high amounts of protein or less than 1,200 calories a day will almost certainly need supplementation. Athletes, too, can use extra nutrients, as they use more energy than the average person. Your doctor may prescribe supplements to counteract medications or illnesses that interfere with vitamin absorption.

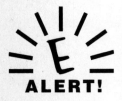

Supplements can be overdosed. Overdose of iron from vitamin supplements is the leading cause of poisoning death in children under the age of six. Keep your vitamins, and all your medications, well out of the reach of children.

If you feel you fit into one of these groups, and you may benefit from vitamin supplements, it is still a good idea to consult a physician.

If you feel you need a supplement because you eat poorly, be sure to choose one that has 100 percent of the RDI for at least ten essential nutrients. Supplements are required to list all of the ingredients and quantities in the supplement facts panel, not simply with the ingredients, even if there is no RDI. This is good news for consumers interested in knowing what they are about to swallow.

Chapter 5

All about Minerals

Minerals are organic chemical elements that, like vitamins, you need in small amounts for growth and metabolism. Like vitamins, they help in the formation of enzymes and hormones, and you get them from the food you eat. This chapter explains the details of minerals and what kinds of foods you should eat to get the minerals you need.

The Main Minerals

Minerals are not as easily destroyed by overcooking or improper handling as vitamins. They are absorbed through your intestines, and transported throughout the body by blood or proteins. These elements can be stored in various forms, so toxicity is more serious. In fact, megadosing of minerals can be quite dangerous. Scientists are still learning about minerals, especially the trace minerals. Supplements are rarely needed, with the exception of iron, which is a very common deficiency.

Science has subdivided minerals into those you need more than 100 milligrams per day of, and what are called trace minerals, those you need less than 100 milligrams a day of.

Calcium

This is the most abundant mineral in the body. You store 98 percent of it in your bones, 1 percent in your teeth, and the last 1 percent circulates around in your blood. It is also extremely common for people to be deficient. Women are prone to deficiency, typically getting only about half of what they need from their regular diet.

Calcium is a crucial element in the normal formation of teeth and bones. With healthy amounts of calcium, human bone growth occurs naturally until middle age, at which time normal bone loss begins. Calcium deficiency limits growth throughout the early years, making adult bones thin and brittle. The effect can be slowed when calcium intake is increased.

Calcium also helps muscles contract and is needed for the production of enzymes and hormones involved in digestion and the conversion of nutrients into energy. It works with vitamin D to regulate blood calcium levels, and it helps blood clot.

Milk is the best source of calcium, but not the only one. Broccoli, kale, spinach, beans, and nuts are all excellent sources. Calcium can also be found fortified in many foods, including cereal, orange juice, and bread.

Calcium absorption can also be inhibited by certain drugs, including cortisone and other steroids, cholesterol-lowering drugs, thyroid drugs, antacids, alcohol, and tobacco.

Phosphorus

This mineral is found in all food, and the average diet gets plenty. It works together with calcium to strengthen your bones and teeth. Like calcium, phosphorus circulates in the bloodstream and goes where it's needed, releasing energy from fat, protein, and carbohydrates. It also contributes to genetic material.

Like calcium, phosphorus is available in milk, as well as meat, poultry, fish eggs, beans, and whole grains. Phosphoric acid is also used in the production of soda pop. There are no good plant sources for phosphorus.

Magnesium

Magnesium is part of the pigment chlorophyll, found in green plants, including spinach and other green leafy vegetables. It can also be found in nuts, beans, and milk.

This mineral is in every tissue, and is necessary in the creation of energy-converting enzymes. It is also used in the formation of bones and teeth. Magnesium is used in the prevention of heart rhythm problems and high blood pressure. It is also thought to prevent migraines and premenstrual syndrome.

Potassium, Sodium, and Chloride: The Electrolytes

Collectively, potassium, sodium, and chloride are referred to as the electrolytes. These are electrically charged minerals that dissolve in body fluid. They carry nutrients in and out of the cells, help send messages along the nerves, and control blood pressure. They are found throughout the body dissolved in water. When you excrete liquids, your electrolytes need to be replaced.

Potassium is found in all living cells. A well-balanced diet contains lots of potassium from several sources, but certain foods are particularly high in potassium, including potatoes, legumes, prunes, and avocados. Sodium and chloride are minerals that you get plenty of in everyday foods, because they are found in table salt. In fact, you probably get too much. They are not just in the shaker, but in prepared foods too.

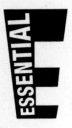

Potassium is found within the cells. Together, sodium and chloride remain outside the cells in fluid. To be in balance, sodium and chloride intake should never be higher than that of potassium. A healthy intake that keeps fluids in balance is considered to be five parts potassium to one part sodium and chloride. If that ration changes, high blood pressure is the result. High blood pressure leads to heart disease, kidney disease, and stroke. Potassium exists in almost every food, but since most people overconsume salt, they need to supplement potassium to stay in balance.

Chloride itself is also part of hydrochloric acid, which is the acid in your stomach that aids digestion and kills bad bacteria. It's not a mineral you need to worry about, though. Since you get plenty of salt in your diet, you are getting enough chloride.

Sodium and Your Family's Health

What is commonly called table salt is sodium chloride (NaCl). It is a combination of the two minerals sodium and chloride, in a 40:60 ratio. You need both minerals, but only in very small quantities. They occur naturally in most foods, but you get the majority of your sodium from manufactured food products. Canned soups and vegetables, condiments, baked goods, chips, and other snack foods are loaded with added salt. It is used in preserving, stabilizing, and flavoring.

As an electrolyte, sodium is essential to keep your body fluids in balance, regulate your blood pressure, spark nerve impulses, relax muscles, and digest proteins and carbohydrates.

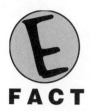

Salt was historically a hot commodity, difficult to obtain and, therefore, quite expensive. It can be harvested from sea water or rock deposits left from ancient seas. From the ocean, salt water is dried by the sun in shallow pools. Mined salt (halite), also known as rock salt, grows in isometric crystals and is very hard.

How Much Salt?

There is no recommended amount of sodium, because people are in no danger of deficiency. Modern Americans consume 4,000 to 6,000 mg of salt every day. The recommended limit of salt is 2,400 mg (just under 1 teaspoon), but your body only needs about 400 mg a day (less than ¼ teaspoon).

Excessive sodium intake can be problematic. Occasionally eating too much sodium is not uncommon, but most of it is excreted in sweat and urine, with the help of your kidneys. You may have experienced a bloated feeling after a particularly salty meal. You most certainly experienced the thirst that follows. Thirst is your body's attempt to regulate fluid balance by sending water to the cells, commonly referred to as water retention. The craving is how the body tells you to drink up.

Sodium and High Blood Pressure

When the kidneys don't work properly to rid the body of excess sodium, a swelling in your feet and legs occurs, known as edema. Excessive sodium intake is a contributing factor to osteoporosis, as well as high blood pressure, also known as hypertension.

As blood flows through your arteries, pressure is created against the arterial wall. If sodium is not eliminated it accumulates in the blood. Water is added to compensate for the imbalance and blood volume increases, leading to high blood pressure. High blood pressure, or hypertension, is a result of too much pressure being placed on the arterial wall.

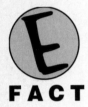

FACT

Your blood pressure is given with two numbers. The systolic pressure (pressure from beating) is the top number, and the diastolic pressure (from relaxing) is the bottom number. The goal is a blood pressure of 120/80. Blood pressure is considered normal if the systolic pressure is 130 or below, and the diastolic pressure is 85 or below. You have high blood pressure from 130–140/85–90, and hypertension above that.

Hypertension is considered a risk factor in coronary artery disease, kidney disease, and stroke. Although not a direct result of sodium intake, elevated sodium levels in combination with other risk factors, including age, heredity, obesity, smoking, alcohol consumption, and limited physical activity can lead to these problems.

Hidden Sodium in Your Diet

Salt has been used in food preservation since ancient times. Just as salt dehydrates you, so too does it dehydrate meat and vegetables. When moisture is removed from foods, bacteria cannot multiply. This process is called curing, and it is an ancient technique used to preserve such foods as meat, fish, vegetables, and olives.

Salt is found in such traditionally cured foods today, including processed meats, capers, anchovies, and cheese. But salt is present in some not-so-obvious foods as well. Condiments, such as ketchup and mustard, are loaded with sodium. Baking soda, baking powder, MSG, and items like Worcestershire and soy sauce have a lot of sodium, too. Breakfast cereal, baked beans, sandwich bread, and ready-made sauces are typically high. Even soft water from your faucet contains sodium. Many chefs prefer kosher salt, which gets its name from its use in the koshering process of meats. Koshering requires that all fluids be extracted from an animal before it is consumed. The larger crystals dissolve more slowly, extracting more fluids from the meat. Kosher salt has no additives, which gives it a cleaner, less-metallic taste.

Table salt is usually iodized. Potassium iodide is added as a dietary supplement to prevent iodine deficiency, a major cause of goiter and cretinism. Most table salt has a water-absorbing additive to keep it from clumping, and some manufacturers add fluoride as well. Before you give up and move to the wilderness, compare labels. The sodium level of a particular product varies by manufacturer. What's more, today there are a wide range of lower sodium options.

Decreasing Your Sodium Intake

If you are concerned about your sodium intake, you have several options. Simply cutting back slowly is probably the best course of action. Unless you have serious hypertension and your doctor has instructed you to quit cold turkey, cut back slowly and let your taste buds become accustomed to the flavor of the foods themselves, not the salted foods.

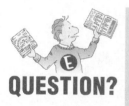

QUESTION?

How can I easily cut back on my salt intake?
First of all, taste your food before you salt it. You may find it tastes fine as it is! Also, do not salt your food as you cook it. Instead, use only the salt on the table. You'll add less overall, and you'll notice it more. Another trick for reducing salt intake is to abandon the salt shaker in favor of the old-fashioned salt cellar. These are small covered containers with a tiny spoon. You have more control over what you use, and you'll use less.

Check the labels of the foods you regularly buy, then choose lower sodium replacements. Salt substitutes are another option, unless you have a sensitivity to potassium. Most substitutes replace at least a portion of sodium chloride with potassium chloride.

Keep track of your daily intake. Nutrition fact panels have made it easy. Total up the daily value percentage of sodium in the foods you consume each day, and try to keep it at or below 100 percent for the day. Check out the recipes at the end of this chapter for some delicious salt substitutes.

Trace Minerals

There are many minerals in the body that science is just beginning to understand. You may be surprised to know that you've got gold, silver, and even arsenic floating around inside your body. The purpose of many of these minerals is still a mystery. Scientists know you need them, but they don't always know why. There are, however, a few of these minerals that are well understood.

Iron

Humans are not often deficient in minerals, except for iron. Iron is a crucial element in each red blood cell. Each molecule of hemoglobin has four iron atoms attached. The quantity of iron determines the quantity of oxygen in the rest of the body. Oxygen attaches to the iron and is carried in the blood to where it is needed. There, it is swapped with carbon dioxide and returned to the lungs where it is exhaled. Too little iron means too few red blood cells. This results in anemia, shortness of breath, fatigue, and paleness.

Deficiency occurs long before symptoms are noticeable. It is common in adult and teenage women (due to the menstrual cycle), and those that lose an excessive amount of blood through surgery or accident. Anyone with poor diet, including picky kids, extreme dieters, and the elderly with loss of appetite, are at risk for deficiency. Vitamin C is important for the absorption of iron, so those with low C intake are also at risk for deficiency. Good sources of iron include meat and poultry, prunes, and oysters, as well as spinach, legumes, and molasses. Another good way to get iron is to cook in it. Food cooked in cast iron absorbs the iron, especially if the food is acidic.

Zinc

Thousands of proteins in your body contain zinc, and it is crucial to the formation of enzymes and hormones, wound healing, DNA synthesis, and a healthy immune system. Normal growth relies on zinc, as it helps utilize proteins, fat, and carbohydrates.

Zinc is found in beans, nuts, and seeds, but the zinc in animal protein is absorbed at a higher rate. Deficiency is rare, but is sometimes found in vegetarians. A vegetarian diet is not simply lacking in meat. It is commonly high in fiber. Excessive fiber binds to zinc and blocks absorption, which can cause various problems.

Selenium

This mineral is an important component of the enzymes that form antioxidants. Working in conjunction with vitamin E, it protects cells from the damage of free radicals. It also plays a role in cell growth and the healthy functioning of the thyroid gland and immune system. The antioxidant and immune system functions of selenium are being studied in relationship to cancer and HIV/AIDS. Seafood is especially rich in selenium, as is meat and poultry. Smaller amounts can be found in grains and nuts. The exception is the Brazil nut, which has the highest levels of selenium of all foods.

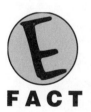

FACT

The first known instance of selenium toxicity was recorded by Marco Polo, who noticed his horses were sloughing layers off of their hooves when they grazed in one particular area of China. That area is now known to have elevated levels of selenium in the soil.

Copper

Copper helps make enzymes that function in energy production. It helps form collagen, connective tissues that support bones, teeth, and muscles. It keeps your arteries flexible, and insulates your nerves. Because copper helps in the absorption of iron, it is crucial in the formation of hemoglobin.

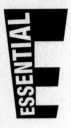

It is said that arthritis sufferers can find relief by wearing copper bracelets. It could be the placebo effect, or it could be that these folks are copper deficient. The ancient Egyptians, Romans, Persians, and Aztecs had many medicinal applications for copper.

Good sources of copper include shellfish, organ meat, legumes, avocados, whole grains, and nuts. Deficiency is rarely caused by diet, but it is sometimes seen as a genetic condition. Toxicity is uncommon, but can cause nausea and damage to the nervous system.

Iodine

This mineral is needed to form the thyroid hormone called thyroxin, which regulates metabolism, or how fast energy from food is used. In general, metabolism refers to a set of reactions that occur in living cells, allowing them to grow, maintain their structure, and react to situations that occur in their environment. But when people speak of their metabolism, they are referring to the way their body burns energy to maintain itself.

Iodine deficiency results in a condition known as hypothyroidism, which is a shortage of thyroid hormone. The body slows the rate at which calories are burned, and in response, the thyroid tries to make more hormone. In doing so, the thyroid swells into a lump known as a goiter.

Iodine is found in seafood and seaweed. Because of low levels of iodine in the Midwestern U.S. soil, and a lack of seafood in the diet, instances of goiters were common in that area. The conditions disappeared in the 1920s when iodine was first added to table salt.

Chromium

This mineral is important in the balance of blood sugar levels, working with insulin to take glucose from the blood to the body cells. Without it, insulin is blocked and blood sugar level is raised. It is also important in the metabolism of fats and proteins. Chromium has been used by bodybuilders and dieters as a way to lose weight and add muscle, and it has been touted as a treatment for diabetes. Such effects have been studied, but have never been proven.

Good sources of chromium include whole grains and lean beef. Brewer's yeast is the most potent source. Only about 2 percent of the chromium you eat is absorbed. Vitamins C and B_3 can help absorption, but most is excreted. When chromium is excreted by excessive sweating, common with extreme exercise, deficiency can occur. Diets with excessive sugar and fat may not include sufficient chromium to balance blood sugar and are therefore deficient. Symptoms include high blood cholesterol, increased arterial plaque, and high blood pressure. Toxicity is rare.

Fluoride

Fluoride is a mineral that your body does not need, but it helps fight tooth decay by hardening tooth enamel. In cities that add fluoride to the water supply, instances of cavities are reduced as much as 40 percent. People that use fluoride toothpaste increase their protection even more. Fluoride is also shown to work in conjunction with calcium, phosphorus, magnesium, and vitamin D to strengthen bones, and it may help in the fight against osteoporosis. Bottled water is not a significant fluoride source.

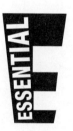

Insulin is a hormone, produced in the pancreas, that makes blood sugar available to your cells as the basic food source. Without insulin, cells cannot access the calories contained within the glucose you ingest.

Mineral Quantities

Following is an easy-to-use list of the minerals, their functions, sources, and the recommended daily intakes. The measurements are listed in various forms because there is not one standard unit, especially for such small amounts.

Mineral Reference Chart

Mineral	RDI	Major Functions	Best Food Sources
Calcium	1,000 mg	strengthens bones, teeth, muscle contraction, and energy conversion	milk, broccoli, green leafy vegetables
Phosphorus	1,000 mg	strengthens bones and teeth, energy conversion, maintains good muscle and nerve function	milk, meat, fish, poultry, beans, grains
Magnesium	400 mg	strengthens bones and teeth, energy conversion, maintains healthy blood pressure	leafy greens, nuts, milk
Iron	18 mg	element of hemoglobin, prevents anemia	meat, poultry, prunes, oysters, molasses
Zinc	15 mg	wound healing, formation of hormones, enzymes, and DNA	meat, beans, nuts, seeds
Selenium	70 mg	antioxidant, healthy thyroid gland and immune system	Brazil nuts, meat, fish, poultry
Copper	2 mg	formation of hemoglobin, collagen, and energy production	shellfish, organ meat, legumes, avocados
Iodine	150 mcg	proper functioning of thyroid gland	seafood, seaweed, iodized salt
Chromium	150 mcg	regulates blood sugar level, metabolism of fat and protein	whole grains, beef, brewer's yeast

Salt-Substitute Recipes

Here are some natural alternatives to salt and salty condiments that you can make at home and keep in your pantry for everyday meals.

Herb Salt Substitute

These herbs can simply be stirred together, but to really blend the flavors, grind them up. They'll pass through a shaker better this way too.

Combine all ingredients in a large bowl and stir together. Working in batches, pulverize in a coffee grinder. Use a funnel to fill a shaker, or store it in an airtight container at room temperature.

Weird Coffee

Coffee grinders are the superior tool for grinding spices. But be sure you have one just for spices. If you use it for coffee beans later, you'll be unpleasantly surprised by the flavor of your joe.

MAKES ABOUT ½ CUP

160 calories
4 g fat
31 g carbohydrates
5 g protein
15 mg sodium
11 g fiber

INGREDIENTS
1 tablespoon cayenne pepper
1 tablespoon onion powder
1 tablespoon garlic powder
1 tablespoon dried savory
1 tablespoon dried thyme
1 tablespoon dried oregano
1 tablespoon dried sage
1 tablespoon nutmeg
1 tablespoon crushed black pepper
Grated zest of 1 lemon

Salt-Free Ketchup

MAKES ABOUT 1 QUART

1,060 calories
33 g fat
202 g carbohydrates
12 g protein
55 mg sodium
16 g fiber

INGREDIENTS

2 tablespoons peanut oil
1 large yellow onion, minced
8 cloves garlic, minced
8 large Roma tomatoes, diced
½ cup honey
½ cup cider vinegar
2 cinnamon sticks, crushed
½ teaspoon whole cloves
1 teaspoon allspice
1 teaspoon celery seed
1 tablespoon dry mustard
1 tablespoon paprika

Once you make your own ketchup, you'll have a hard time going back to the bottled stuff.

1. Heat oil in a large saucepan over medium heat. Add onion and garlic and cook, stirring, until golden brown.

2. Add tomatoes, honey, vinegar, cinnamon sticks, and cloves and stir to moisten. Bring to a boil, reduce heat, and simmer 20–30 minutes, stirring occasionally.

3. Add allspice, celery seed, mustard, and paprika and cook another 5 minutes. Remove from heat and cool.

4. Working in batches, run sauce through a food processor, blender, or food mill until it becomes a smooth puree. Strain through a wire-mesh strainer back into the saucepan and place over high heat. Cook, stirring continuously, until the sauce reaches desired thickness, about 10–15 minutes. Chill before serving. Store refrigerated for 2–3 days, or freeze for several weeks.

Citrus Salt Substitute

Citrus zest is loaded with flavor. The essential oils are concentrated where the bright color is and will stay there until released by grating or grinding. Peeling the zest with a peeler keeps as much of the oil in the zest as possible until you are ready to release it among the rest of the spices in this recipe.

1. Preheat oven to 200°F. Using a vegetable peeler, carefully remove the brightly colored zest from the lemons, oranges, and limes. (Do not peel off the white pith underneath.) Lay the zests in a single layer on a baking sheet. Bake 15–30 minutes, until dry and crisp. Alternatively, zests can be placed in the hot sunshine.

2. Combine zests and remaining ingredients in a large bowl and stir together. Working in batches, pulverize in a coffee grinder. Use a funnel to fill a shaker, or store it in an airtight container at room temperature.

MAKES ABOUT ½ CUP

320 calories
3 g fat
81 g carbohydrates
8 g protein
15 mg sodium
21 g fiber

INGREDIENTS
2 lemons
2 oranges
2 limes
2 tablespoons minced fresh rosemary
2 tablespoons ground black pepper
2 tablespoons lemon verbena (if available)
1 tablespoon celery seed
½ teaspoon white pepper
½ teaspoon dill weed
½ teaspoon dried thyme
¾ teaspoon sour salt (powdered citric acid)

Garlic Salt Substitute

The tangy addition of dill and celery seed really sets this blend apart.

Combine all ingredients in a large bowl and stir together. Working in batches, pulverize in a coffee grinder. Use a funnel to fill a shaker, or store it in an airtight container at room temperature.

Salt Warning
Be sure you buy garlic powder and not garlic salt. As the name implies, garlic salt is loaded with sodium. Onion salt is out there too, so beware.

MAKES ABOUT ½ CUP

140 calories
1.5 g fat
31 g carbohydrates
6 g protein
15 mg sodium
5 g fiber

INGREDIENTS
3 tablespoons granulated garlic
3 tablespoons dried onion
Grated zest of 1 lemon
1 teaspoon dried thyme
1 teaspoon dried rosemary
1 teaspoon dill seed
1 teaspoon celery seed

Salt-Free Tomato Sauce

**MAKES ABOUT
1 QUART**

670 calories
33 g fat
88 g carbohydrates
14 g protein
70 mg sodium
26 g fiber

INGREDIENTS
*2 tablespoons olive oil
1 large yellow onion, diced
3 cloves garlic
¼ cup dried basil
¼ cup dried oregano
2 tablespoons ground fennel
    seed
1 tablespoon red chili flakes
¼ cup balsamic vinegar
Zest and juice of 1 lemon
8 large Roma tomatoes,
    diced*

*Use this sauce for pasta, pizza, or as the base
for hearty winter soups and stews.*

1. Heat oil in a large saucepan over medium heat. Add onion, garlic, and cook, stirring, until golden brown.

2. Add basil, oregano, fennel, and chili flakes and stir to moisten.

3. Add vinegar, lemon juice and zest, and tomatoes. Bring to a boil, reduce heat, and simmer 20–30 minutes, stirring occasionally, until flavors are well blended, and sauce is reduced to desired thickness. Cool completely.

4. Working in batches, run sauce through a food processor, blender, or food mill until it becomes a smooth puree. Strain through a wire-mesh strainer. Use immediately, refrigerate for 2–3 days, or freeze for up to a month.

Salt-Free Barbecue Sauce

*This sauce can go toe to toe with any salty barbecue sauce. It's
sweet and tangy, just like the best barbeque chefs' recipes.*

1. Heat oil in a large saucepan over medium heat. Add onion and garlic.
   Cook, stirring, until golden brown.

2. Add honey, molasses, and vinegar and stir to warm through.

3. Add powdered chilies, mustard, cayenne pepper, celery seed, and
   water. Bring to a boil, then reduce heat and simmer for 14–20 minutes, stirring occasionally, until flavors are well blended and sauce is
   reduced to desired thickness. Use immediately or store refrigerated for
   up to a week.

MAKES ABOUT 3 CUPS

1,550 calories
39 g fat
314 g carbohydrates
13 g protein
100 mg sodium
15 g fiber

INGREDIENTS
*2 tablespoons peanut oil
1 large yellow onion, diced
6 cloves garlic, minced
½ cup honey
½ cup molasses
½ cup cider vinegar
¼ cup powdered red chilies
2 tablespoons powdered
    mustard
1 tablespoon cayenne pepper
1 tablespoon ground cumin
1 teaspoon celery seed
2 cups water*

Salt-Free Oven Fries

*These fries are not only salt free, they are fat free and have no
refined sugar! Don't tell anyone though. They'll never know.*

1. Preheat oven to 450°F.

2. In a large bowl, combine potatoes and seasoning. Add egg whites and
   toss together until well coated.

3. Spread into one layer on a nonstick baking sheet or roasting pan.
   Bake 10 minutes, remove from oven, and stir briefly. Return to oven
   for another 10 minutes, and stir again. Repeat this for another 30–40
   minutes, until potatoes are crisp, brown, and tender. Serve immediately
   with Salt-Free Ketchup (page 58).

SERVES 6

155 calories
< 1 g fat
34 g carbohydrates
5 g protein
31 mg sodium
4 g fiber

INGREDIENTS
*3 large russet potatoes,
    sliced in ¼-inch sticks
2 tablespoons Garlic Salt
    Substitute (page 59)
2 egg whites*

Chapter 6

The Power of Protein

Protein is a vital component of living cells. Its general function is to build and maintain the body. Its many functions throughout the body are so crucial that without it, malnutrition is a serious risk. Luckily, protein is not hard to obtain, even for vegetarians. There are a multitude of sources that fit easily into any cuisine. In this chapter you will explore protein and learn interesting ways to add it to your menus.

The Role of Protein in a Healthy Diet

Protein builds and maintains muscles, organs, connective tissues, skin, bones, teeth, blood, and your DNA (deoxyribonucleic acid). It helps the body heal when it is sick, wounded, or depleted. Without it, even mild exercise would weaken you to the point of exhaustion.

Protein contributes to the formation of enzymes. Almost all reactions that occur in the body, such as digestion, require enzymes. Enzymes are catalysts to these reactions, increasing the rate at which they occur.

There is protein in your blood, called antibodies. They serve as your body's immune responders. They bind with and fight foreign invaders, like bacteria or toxins. Protein is found in hormones, your body's chemical messengers. Hormones help regulate the body's activities, maintaining balance, or *homeostasis*.

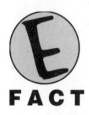

Soy, amaranth, and quinoa are the only plant species that contain complete protein. Soy is available in many forms, including beans, tofu, milk, and supplements. Amaranth and quinoa are grains available in health food stores, and many mainstream markets.

Amino Acids

Protein is composed of twenty amino acids. These acids link together in chains to form the variety of proteins your body needs. The length and shape of the chain determines the protein's structure. Of the twenty amino acids, eleven of them are made by your body. These eleven acids are called *nonessential* because you do not need to consume them. The remaining nine amino acids are called *essential*, and it is important that you eat these every day. Getting all nine essential amino acids is not hard, especially if you eat meat. Animal foods (which include meat, eggs, and dairy) contain the largest concentration of protein. Animal protein is considered *complete*, because it contains all nine essential amino acids.

Plant foods also contain proteins, but few plants contain complete protein. This is one of the challenges of vegetarianism, because to stay healthy one must consume enough foods with the right mixture of amino acids. It sounds complicated, but grains, nuts, and legumes contain the proteins that are not found in other plants, so adding a variety of these to your diet does the trick.

Plant foods eaten in combination to create complete protein are called *complementary proteins*. When these foods are eaten over the course of a day, protein intake is complete. Protein derived from complementary plant proteins is considered a healthy alternative, and by many people, a superior one. Eating such combinations of plant foods not only completes the protein, but also provides other nutrients vital to good health as well, most notably fiber, vitamins, and minerals. And most plants do all that without saturated fat.

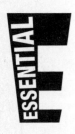

Eating complementary protein means consuming both beans and grains every day. The beans can be pinto, kidney, black, lentils, garbanzo, split peas, or peanuts. Grains should be whole, including brown rice, whole-wheat pasta, bread, crackers, or tortillas. Sesame seeds also complement the protein of beans.

Cooking Protein

Cooked protein is also referred to as *denatured*. When denatured, protein changes its structure and stops functioning. In denaturation, the amino acids loosen, recoil, and tighten, which changes the appearance, texture, and flavor of the protein. If you watch an egg being cooked, you can see the denaturation happen within a minute or two as the albumen turns white.

Cooking protein does not necessarily require heat. Acid will denature protein, as it does in the Latin American dish seviche, in which seafood is marinated in lime. Salt is used to cook protein in cured meats, like ham, sausages, and salt cod. Pickled meats combine acid and salt for a double-whammy cooking method. Even agitation can denature protein, as in the whipping of eggs. In this case prolonged agitation changes the egg's structure, making it safe to eat. Meringue demonstrates this effect on the egg white, while yolks and whole eggs get this treatment in mayonnaise and emulsified salad dressings, like those used in Caesar salad.

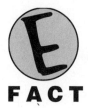

FACT

Denaturation of protein doesn't happen only in the kitchen. You've also seen it at your last visit to the beach. The waves break onto the sand, the tide rolls in and out, and that motion denatures the proteins in the sea water, creating sea foam.

Choosing Your Protein

People in the United States overconsume animal protein. To stay healthy and rebuild muscle the average adult needs only five to six ounces of complete protein each day. But a typical American diet consists of bacon and eggs for breakfast, a meat-filled sandwich for lunch, and a dinner featuring meat as its focus. A healthy family needs a healthy diet of lean protein in moderation. Animal proteins are higher in fat and particularly saturated fat, which in turn makes them high in cholesterol. Plant foods, however, contain no cholesterol, less fat (in the form of plant oil), and lots of fiber.

Eating too little protein is not healthy, but neither is eating too much. Overeating protein does not build extra muscle. The protein your body does not utilize is stored as fat.

Meat

While *meat* is a common generic term meaning flesh, to chefs it refers specifically to four-legged domesticated animals. This includes mainly beef, lamb, and pork. Lamb is just now becoming popular in America, and pork is gaining in popularity as a lean meat option. But by far, the favorite meat in the United States is beef.

Historically, the cow's size made it more valuable as a draft animal than a source of food. The logistics of slaughtering such a large animal were daunting. Preservation methods revolved around salting, and such methods were not very sophisticated. Unless there was a real crowd to feed, lamb was a more popular choice. But modern Americans love cows. They no longer harness the strength of the cow, but the meat, milk, and hide easily make it the world's most important domesticated animal.

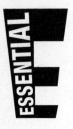

Worldwide food consumption statistics show 65 percent of protein comes from plants. When looking only at U.S. food consumption, however, only about 30 percent of protein comes from plants. It is essential for your good health to obtain more of your weekly protein from plants.

Choosing Beef

Beef and veal are readily available in modern supermarkets, and for the most part, quality is high. The United States Department of Agriculture (USDA) grades meat for consumption based on muscle-to-bone and fat-to-muscle ratios. Beef grades, from best to worse, are prime, choice, and select. Lesser grades, used mainly for processed meat products, include standard, commercial, and utility. Grades are stamped in purple on the outer carcass of the animal, and are usually prominently advertised by retailers, especially when the grade is high.

Beef cows are taken to market at between eighteen and twenty-four months of age. Before that time it is considered veal. Veal is a male dairy cow between sixteen and eighteen months of age. Veal grades, from best to worse, are prime, choice, good, standard, and utility.

The Disadvantages of Meat

Meat is generally considered a high-fat protein choice. Of course, usually fat means flavor. In today's world people appreciate, and even expect, a high level of flavor in their meat, despite full knowledge that saturated fat contributes to coronary artery disease and elevated cholesterol levels.

There are lean cuts available, but even if you cannot see the fat marbled throughout a particular cut, the saturated fat is still present within the muscle cells. When meat is heated, the fat melts and penetrates the muscle. So even if you do not eat the visible fat on a steak, you are consuming saturated fat.

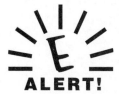

ALERT!

A leaner diet is healthier, not just for your body, but for the planet. Today, herds are a burden on ecosystems. Waste seeps into groundwater and contaminates nearby crops, grazing results in defoliation and erosion, and the United Nations even recognizes livestock as one of the largest contributors of greenhouse gasses. The key to a healthy body and planet is moderation.

This appetite for fatty beef has drastically changed the landscape of modern agriculture. Today cattle is bred and raised to provide the most meat with the least cost. According to the USDA, the average American consumes sixty-seven pounds of beef every year.

A wild cow would naturally consume fiber-rich plants that are unsuitable for human consumption. Today, cows compete with humans for food, consuming grain grown on valuable fertile soil. In the United States half of the water, and 80 percent of the grain harvested, goes to livestock.

Poultry

Poultry is the term used to describe domesticated birds raised for food. In the United States this means mainly chicken and turkey. Duck, while common in Europe and Asia, appears more often on restaurant menus than in your grocery store. Game hens are another form of poultry that appears from time to time.

Whenever possible, buy free-range, organic poultry. Common chickens are raised with profit, not health, in mind. They must be fed antibiotics to fend off disease. They are given growth hormones, which, coupled with lack of exercise, makes them so fat they cannot move. In addition, the food they are fed is grown with artificial fertilizers and chemical pesticides.

Choosing Your Bird

There are several organic options available in most stores, including *organic, free-range*, and *natural birds*. Free-range chickens have more flavor because they are allowed to exercise a bit more. Natural birds contain nothing synthetic, no preservatives or artificial flavoring or colorings, but standards permit antibiotics and hormone use. Organic birds are fed grains that have not been exposed to chemicals and pesticides. They may not be treated with antibiotics or drugs, and must be allowed to go outside and exercise.

Kosher chickens are organic and free range, and are processed under strict supervision of a rabbi. They are also soaked in salty brine, which gives them a unique flavor.

When shopping for chickens, frugal cooks know that whole chickens are always less expensive than cut-up parts. But unless you possess good butchering skills, it can be worth paying a little more. Keep in mind that chicken fat occurs in and around the skin, and is easy to remove.

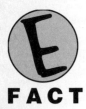

FACT

Mollusks are further categorized. *Gastropods* are one-shelled mollusks, such as abalone and limpets, two animals eaten extensively in seaside nations around the world. In the United States we are more accustomed to *bivalves*, which are mollusks with two shells and a hinge, like the oyster. *Cephalopods,* which include squid and octopus, are shellfish too, although they have tentacles instead of shells.

Seafood

Seafood is the most abundant source of protein there is. Consider all the varieties, around the world, and it's an immense category of food. Narrowed down to its basic parts, the world of seafood is easy to navigate. Seafood is a name given to all marine animals caught or raised for food. This includes both fresh and saltwater species. People tend to condense them all into a general category of fish, but there are many subcategories.

Fish Groups

Fish is first divided into two basic types: *finfish* and *shellfish*. There are two kinds of finfish: flat fish and round fish. The flat fish, which include flounder, halibut, and sole, skim along the bottom of the sea. Round fish (which only appear round if they are swimming straight toward you) are found in both fresh and salt water. The fresh water fish have much smaller bones than their larger, oceangoing cousins. Shellfish are also separated into two categories: *mollusks*, such as mussels and clams, and *crustaceans*, which includes crabs, lobsters, crayfish, and shrimp.

Choosing Fish

If you are lucky enough to live near the sea, you will likely have an abundance of fish at your market. Further inland, your fish selection may be more limited. Luckily, frozen fish today are of very high quality, as they are flash-frozen on board the ship that caught them.

When buying frozen fish, be sure it is free of ice, which is a sign that it has been defrosted and refrozen. It should have a natural shape, with only a light coating of frost. Defrost frozen fish slowly, twenty-four to thirty-six hours in the refrigerator is best. Place defrosting fish in a colander or perforated pan to separate the runoff juices. Smaller pieces can be cooked frozen.

When buying fresh fish, be sure that all you smell is fresh, oceany fish. If the smell is offputting, don't buy it. When you get it home, store it in the fridge loosely covered in paper, preferably in a perforated pan to allow juices to drain away. If the fish is stored longer than two to three days, it should be frozen.

Game

Game is the name given to meat that was traditionally hunted. Deer (venison), rabbits, boar, squirrel, and possum are the most common game meats, although anything wild fits the category. Game bird is a subcategory of game, containing such species as pheasant, ostrich, quail, and partridge. Even though many of these animals are raised in captivity today, they are still considered game by virtue of their history and their stronger flavors. Game meats can be prepared in the same manner as domestic meats. Traditionally, the more active muscles required prolonged tenderizing through marinades, and longer, moist-heat cooking methods. But farm-raised game meats can stand fast high heat.

In general, the flavor of wild animal meat is stronger than that of farm animals. These creatures eat a different diet, and get an enormous amount of exercise, which alters the muscle tissue. The taste is often too strong for modern palettes, which are more accustomed to grocery store meat.

Eggs

The nutritional value of eggs cannot be denied. They are loaded with protein and are, as such, used as a measure for other proteins. What's more, they contain almost every essential vitamin and mineral humans need.

The egg yolk contains a high percentage of cholesterol, and people watching their cholesterol should avoid them. But normal, healthy, active humans can, and should, benefit from the incredible egg.

Choosing Your Eggs

When possible, look for organic eggs from free-range chickens. They are regulated to a certain extent by the USDA. No antibiotics or hormones are allowed, and the animals are provided with access to the outdoors. Eggs have a tremendous shelf life. By the time they get to your grocer, they are one or two weeks old. When you get them home they will last in your fridge another three weeks. The shell, which is very porous, allows odor and moisture to pass through. As time passes, the yolk and white become thinner. Thicker, fresher egg whites and yolks are preferable for recipes that require the eggs to be whipped.

Beans

The general term *bean* encompasses several plants and usually refers to the *legume*, a large plant seed found within long pods from the plant family Fabaceae. Soybeans, peas, lentils, and kidney beans are examples of legumes.

When the seeds are dried, they are referred to as pulse. Many beans are only sold in dry form, while some, such as the pea, come both dried and fresh.

Beans are an excellent choice for low-fat protein, with more than twice the amount of protein as grain. Beans are available in dried or canned form. Dried beans take longer to cook, and must first undergo a long soaking to tenderize them. Canned beans are readily available, which makes it easy to add beans into your everyday diet. Common beans available in most markets include adzuki, broad bean, cannellini, chickpeas, fava, kidney, lentil, lima, mung, navy, pea, pinto, runner, soy, and white.

Nuts

Botanically, a nut is a fruit with one seed. The wall of the seed becomes very hard, and the meat of the seed stays very loose within. Walnuts, pecans, hazelnuts, and chestnuts fall into this category. However, in the world of cuisine there are other nuts that do not fit the definition. Peanuts are legumes, the pine nut is a seed from a pine tree, a macadamia nut is a kernel, and the Brazil nut is found inside a fruit capsule.

Nuts have a high oil content, and can easily become rancid if stored improperly. Heat and light increase rancidity, so refrigeration is best for long-term storage. Flavor is greatly altered, and generally improved, by heat. Toasting nuts in an oven yields the best results. Spread them out on a baking sheet and roast at 350°F for 10–15 minutes, until they become fragrant.

Healthy, Protein-Rich Recipes

The following recipes feature low-fat, protein-rich ingredients from each of the categories discussed. Many of the meats are interchangeable, and recipes can easily be adjusted to suit your taste. For instance, if you are not a fan of spicy heat, you can omit the chilies in the Southwestern Grilled Flank Steak Salad.

Southwestern Grilled Flank Steak Salad

SERVES 4

435 calories
33 g fat
25 g carbohydrates
21 g protein
863 mg sodium
8 g fiber

INGREDIENTS

*Juice and zest of 2 limes
    (about 2 tablespoons)
2 cloves garlic, minced
¼ cup fresh cilantro, minced
½ teaspoon kosher salt
½ teaspoon ground black
    pepper
½ cup olive oil
1 (½-pound) grilled flank
    steak, cooled and sliced
    thin
1 cup green onions, chopped
1 (15-ounce) can black beans,
    rinsed
1 red bell pepper, diced
1 Anaheim chili, diced
1 tomato, diced*

*Plan ahead. At your next barbecue, make an extra steak and save
    it for this salad. It's great made with grilled chicken too.*

1. In a large bowl whisk together lime zest and juice, garlic, cilantro, salt, and pepper. Drizzle in oil while whisking.

2. Add steak, onions, beans, bell pepper, chili, and tomato and toss to coat.

3. Cover and chill 1 hour to allow flavors to mingle. Serve chilled.

Finishing Touches

Top each serving with a dollop of homemade guacamole or light sour cream. The added cool creamy moisture will relieve the spicy heat, and it adds a nice textural balance. Or make it even healthier by substituting plain yogurt, seasoned with a touch of cumin. You get all the benefit of calcium without the fat.

Marinated Lamb Shish Kebabs

The name shish kebab means "skewer of roasted meat," and similar dishes are found throughout Eastern Europe, the Middle East, and Asia. Both metal and wooden skewers work fine, but be sure to soak wooden ones in warm water for at least thirty minutes so they won't ignite.

1. Mix together wine, olive oil, Worcestershire, vinegar, thyme, and salt. Combine with cubed meat in a large zipper-top food storage bag. Zip tight and massage marinade into the lamb. Refrigerate for at least 1 hour or overnight.

2. Preheat grill on high heat. Skewer the meat and vegetables separately to ensure even cooking.

3. Brush the vegetables with olive oil. Grill vegetables off direct heat, turning frequently until they are golden brown, about 10 minutes.

4. Grill meat kebabs over direct high heat for 5–10 minutes, turning frequently to brown evenly.

5. Remove meat and vegetables from skewers onto platters. Serve kebabs with a big platter of rice, or couscous.

Ancient Techniques

This dish is said to have been originated by Turkish soldiers roasting meat on their swords. But it is likely that the concept originated much earlier. The method allows portions of food to be cooked over a very small fire.

SERVES 4

1,175 calories
77 g fat
31 g carbohydrates
60 g protein
850 mg sodium
13 g fiber

INGREDIENTS
1 (750 ml) bottle red wine (about 3½ cups)
2 tablespoons olive oil
1 tablespoon Worcestershire sauce
1 tablespoon red wine vinegar
1 tablespoon dried thyme
1 teaspoon kosher salt
2 pounds lamb shoulder, cut into 2-inch cubes
12 skewers
1 pint cherry tomatoes
8 ounces small button mushrooms
2 small zucchinis, sliced into 2-inch wheels
2 small Chinese eggplants, sliced into 2-inch wheels
1 large yellow onion, quartered
½ cup olive oil

Turkey Burgers

SERVES 6

347 calories
14 g fat
21 g carbohydrates
31 g protein
542 mg sodium
1 g fiber

INGREDIENTS
2 pounds ground turkey
½ teaspoon kosher salt
½ teaspoon black pepper
6 large hamburger buns,
   toasted

The turkey burger is a true American original. With less fat than ground beef, it is significantly healthier than a burger made from beef, cutting about 200 calories, and 7 grams of fat.

1. Divide hamburger into six equal portions. Work the meat in your hand, patting out the air and compacting the meat. Form portions into ½-inch thick discs and make a hole in the very center of each with your finger.

2. Preheat the grill on high heat. Place burgers over direct heat and cook 2–3 minutes with the lid closed. Open the lid, flip burgers, and cook another 2–3 minutes. If the burgers do not come off the grill easily for the first flip, close the lid and cook another minute. Season with salt and pepper, then serve on a bun. Let your guests doctor them up with sliced tomatoes, onions, lettuce, pickles, Thousand Island dressing, ketchup, mustard, and mayonnaise.

Kitchen Tricks
Why put a hole in the center of each patty? This trick keeps the patty from puffing up into a ball on the grill. Another trick for juicy burgers is to resist pressing the burger onto the grill with your spatula, which dries the burger out. With so much less fat than beef, you need all the moisture you can get.

Curried Chicken Stir-Fry

This recipe is best made in a wok, but if you are wok-less, a large sauté pan will do.

1. Combine chicken and curry powder in a large plastic zipper-top bag. Rub spices into meat and refrigerate at least 1 hour, or overnight.

2. Heat peanut oil in a wok over high heat. Add garlic and ginger, stirring quickly to coat with oil.

3. Add marinated chicken and stir continuously for 1 minute.

4. Add carrots, celery, zucchini, squash, and peas and cook 3–5 minutes, stirring, until vegetables are tender, but still bright.

5. Add onions and sesame seeds and toast another minute.

6. Add lime juice and honey and toss to coat.

7. Remove from heat, stir in cilantro, and serve over steamed jasmine rice.

Maximizing Nutrients

Stir-fried vegetables are often sliced at an angle. This exposes more surface area from the heart of the vegetable, allowing it to cook quickly and thoroughly. Remember that heat dissipates nutrients, so faster cooking keeps more nutrients within the vegetable, and more get into you!

SERVES 4

263 calories
12 g fat
25 g carbohydrates
18 g protein
98 mg sodium
7 g fiber

INGREDIENTS
2 boneless, skinless chicken breasts, sliced in ¼-inch strips
2 tablespoons curry powder or paste
2 tablespoons peanut oil
1 clove garlic, sliced
2 tablespoons ginger root, grated
2 medium carrots, sliced
2 stalks celery, sliced
1 zucchini, sliced
2 yellow summer squash, sliced
1 cup snap peas, trimmed
1 cup green onions, chopped
2 tablespoons sesame seeds
Juice of 2 limes (about 1 tablespoon)
1 tablespoon honey
½ cup cilantro, chopped

Mustard Marinated Rabbit

SERVES 4

603 calories
18 g fat
15 g carbohydrates
74 g protein
1,843 mg sodium
< 1 g fiber

INGREDIENTS
1 (3–5 pound) rabbit, cut into
    serving pieces
2 cups white wine
1 cup Dijon mustard
2 bay leaves, crushed
1 teaspoon thyme
3 tablespoons peanut oil
¼ cup cognac or brandy
1 cup chicken stock

Rabbit meat is leaner than most meats, including chicken. It is a well-loved ingredient throughout the world, but has not gained much popularity here in the United States.

1. Combine rabbit, wine, mustard, bay leaves, and thyme in a large plastic zipper-top bag. Rub marinade into the meat and refrigerate for at least 3 hours, or overnight.

2. Heat a large cast iron skillet over high heat. Add peanut oil, remove rabbit from marinade, and brown on all sides.

3. Add marinade, cognac, stock, reduce heat to low, cover and simmer for 1 hour, until tender.

Rabbit Accompaniments
Serve this hearty stew over something grainy, to soak up the tangy sauce. Brown or wild rice make an excellent base, as does quinoa or couscous. Traditionally, such dishes are served over buttered noodles. A healthier version would be whole-wheat noodles tossed in olive oil.

Grilled Tuna Niçoise

You can prepare the topping to this dish up to a day in advance. The added time will intensify the flavors. Remember, when cooking fish of any kind, follow the ten-minutes-per-inch rule: ten minutes of moderate heat for every inch of thickness.

1. Preheat grill on high heat. In a large bowl combine olives, onions, capers, tomatoes, parsley, olive oil, and wine vinegar. Toss together and set aside at room temperature.

2. Coat tuna steaks with lemon juice, salt, pepper, and grill. Cook 5–10 minutes per side, until meat is firm and cooked through. Serve immediately topped with olive mixture.

The Caper Story

Native to the Mediterranean, capers are green buds from a small evergreen bush that are dried and pickled in vinegar brine, or packed in salt. Their flavor is tangy and salty, and they work nicely in acidic dishes like this one. Look for them in the same grocery store aisle as pickles and olives. If you buy the salted version, be sure to rinse the salt off before you use them.

SERVES 4

565 calories
47 g fat
16 g carbohydrates
22 g protein
1,295 mg sodium
3 g fiber

INGREDIENTS

2 cups kalamata olives, pitted
    and halved
1 yellow onion, minced
¼ cup capers
2 tomatoes, chopped
¼ cup fresh parsley, chopped
½ cup olive oil
½ cup red wine vinegar
4 (3-ounce) tuna steaks
½ cup lemon juice
⅛ teaspoon kosher salt
½ teaspoon black pepper

Spinach and Mushroom Frittata

SERVES 6

232 calories
17 g fat
5 g carbohydrates
15 g protein
212 mg sodium
1 g fiber

INGREDIENTS
2 tablespoons olive oil
1 medium yellow onion,
*   diced*
3 cups sliced mushrooms
2 cloves garlic, minced
4 cups chopped fresh
*   spinach*
¼ cup chopped fresh basil
8 eggs
1 cup grated Monterey jack
*   cheese*
1 teaspoon grated nutmeg
Salt and pepper to taste

Frittata is a favorite recipe among chefs and caterers. It can be sliced into any shape and used as a main dish, appetizer, or passed hors d'oeuvre. It tastes great hot or cold and actually improves with age.

1. Preheat oven to 350°F. Coat a casserole dish lightly with pan spray or olive oil.

2. Heat oil in a large sauté pan over medium heat. Add onions and cook until tender.

3. Add mushrooms and garlic and cook until browned.

4. Add spinach and continue cooking until wilted.

5. Remove from heat, add basil, eggs, cheese, nutmeg, salt, and pepper. Transfer to prepared dish. Bake in oven for 30 minutes until firm and golden brown.

Spanish Frittata
Frittata is the Italian name of this open-faced omelet. In Spain a similar dish goes by the name tortilla, and is essentially a potato frittata. The name means "little torta" or "round loaf," and unlike their Mexican counterparts, they are a meal unto themselves.

Venison Stew

Venison is lean and tender, with a distinctive flavor, unlike veal or lamb. If you're not a hunter, you can find venison at gourmet markets, or on the Internet at www.venisonamerica.com.

1. Coat venison evenly with flour and shake off excess. Heat oil in a large cast iron skillet over high heat, then brown meat on all sides. Work in batches if necessary so as not to crowd meat in pan.

2. Add garlic and onion to the meat and sauté 5 minutes.

3. Add tomato paste, thyme, bay leaf, and stock. Bring to a boil, reduce heat to low, cover, and cook at a bare simmer for 1 hour.

4. Add the potatoes and carrots, cover and continue cooking another 30 minutes, until vegetables are tender. Season with salt and pepper before serving with a sprinkle of fresh parsley on top.

Variation on a Theme
You can change the flavor of this stew by replacing part of the stock with red wine, white wine, apple cider, or dark beer (preferably Guinness stout). You can also turn it into a goulash of sorts by adding about ¼ cup of good Hungarian paprika.

SERVES 6

549 calories
9 g fat
58 g carbohydrates
60 g protein
1,620 mg sodium
9 g fiber

INGREDIENTS
1 tablespoon olive oil
2 pounds venison stew meat (shoulder or butt), cut into 1-inch cubes
2 cups whole-wheat flour
1 tablespoon olive oil
2 cloves garlic
1 onion chopped
2 tablespoons tomato paste
1 tablespoon dried thyme
1 bay leaf
6 cups beef stock
2 large russet potatoes, peeled and diced
2 carrots, diced
½ tablespoon kosher salt
½ tablespoon black pepper
2 tablespoons fresh parsley, chopped

Six-Bean Salad

SERVES 8

480 calories
20 g fat
66 g carbohydrates
14 g protein
1,040 mg sodium
14 g fiber

INGREDIENTS
½ cup honey
⅔ cup olive oil
Juice and zest of 6 limes
½ cup white wine vinegar
1 teaspoon kosher salt
1 teaspoon ground black
    pepper
1 red, yellow, or green bell
    pepper, chopped
1 (15-ounce) can kidney
    beans, drained
1 (15-ounce) can yellow wax
    beans, drained
1 (15-ounce) can green string
    beans, drained
1 (15-ounce) can chick peas,
    drained
1 (15-ounce) can cannellini
    beans, drained
1 (15-ounce) can black beans,
    rinsed and drained
1 medium purple onion,
    chopped and soaked in
    cold water for 15–20
    minutes
2 scallions, chopped

This recipe is twice as good as the three-bean version. It's a great choice for picnics because it has no mayonnaise, and can sit out in the sun all day. It actually tastes better when it's at room (or park) temperature.

1. In a large bowl, combine the honey, oil, lime juice, vinegars, and salt and pepper. Mix well to combine.

2. Add the bell pepper, beans, and onions. Toss well to coat with dressing, cover with plastic wrap, and refrigerate at least 2 hours, or overnight.

Taming Onions
Soaking onions in cold water removes the harsh onion oil that causes bad breath. Slice them as needed, and submerge them in ice water while you prepare the rest of your dish. Then, drain them and add them in last. For longer soaks, change the water every hour to get rid of the offensive oils.

Egg Fried Rice

This recipe makes a terrific side dish, lunch, or a light diner. Easy and fast, it can be beefed up (so to speak) with thinly sliced chicken breast, shrimp, or tofu.

1. In a small bowl, mix together eggs, sesame oil, and soy sauce.

2. Heat peanut oil in a sauté pan over high heat. Add rice and fry, stirring, until heated through, about 5 minutes.

3. Add egg mixture and continue stirring to cook eggs, another 2–3 minutes.

4. Add onions and sesame seeds, stir briefly, and serve.

Waste Not, Want Not

This is a great use for leftover rice. In fact, it's an all-around great leftover dish. Add last night's veggies and meat for a filling lunch or dinner. If you plan on making it from the beginning, make it easy on yourself and make the rice ahead of time.

SERVES 4

193 calories
13 g fat
14 g carbohydrates
5 g protein
290 mg sodium
2 g fiber

INGREDIENTS
*2 eggs
2 teaspoons sesame oil
1 tablespoon soy sauce
2 tablespoons peanut oil
1 cup brown rice, cooked and
   cooled
½ cup green onions, chopped
1 tablespoon sesame seeds*

Almond Horchata

This cinnamon-flavored rice drink is a staple throughout Latin America and Spain. It can be found made from rice, barley, and a variety of nuts. Cool and refreshing, it typically appears alongside other aguas frescas made from tamarind, hibiscus, and melon.

SERVES 6

488 calories
16 g fat
80 g carbohydrates
9 g protein
100 mg sodium
4 g fiber

INGREDIENTS
5 cups water
4 cinnamon sticks
1 cup rice
2 cups sliced almonds, toasted
1 cup honey
1 tablespoon vanilla extract
¼ teaspoon kosher salt
4–6 lime wedges

1. Combine water and cinnamon in a large saucepan and bring to a boil over high heat. Reduce heat to low and simmer 15 minutes. Remove from heat and cool to lukewarm.

2. In a blender or food processor pulse rice to a fine powder.

3. Add ground rice and nuts to cinnamon water and steep 1 hour.

4. Add honey, vanilla, and salt, and return to blender. Puree until thick and creamy. Strain through a fine mesh strainer or cheesecloth. Serve over ice with a wedge of lime.

The Perfect Grind
You can grind rice in a food processor, but with only 1 cup to grind, it will likely spin around the outside of the processor bowl, barely hitting the blade. To get the finest possible grind for this amount, use a coffee grinder.

Spiced Nuts

This snack is easy and elegant. It is best made with good quality Italian Parmesan cheese and extra-virgin olive oil.

1. Preheat oven to 375°F.

2. Spread nuts on baking sheet in an even layer. Toast until fragrant and browned, 10–15 minutes. Remove from oven.

3. While hot, toss nuts in olive oil, thyme, pepper, onion, fennel, salt, and Parmesan cheese. Spread out again to cool before serving. Store airtight in the refrigerator or freezer.

Sweet and Spicy
Make Sweet Spiced Nuts by replacing the cheese and spices with ½ cup brown sugar and 1 teaspoon each of cinnamon, nutmeg, ginger, and allspice. Or make them Hot and Spicy by adding ½ teaspoon each of cayenne, white, and black peppers.

SERVES 8–10

625 calories
56 g fat
19 g carbohydrates
22 g protein
247 mg sodium
12 g fiber

INGREDIENTS
4 cups whole, skin-on almonds
3 tablespoons olive oil
1 teaspoon dried thyme
1 teaspoon ground black pepper
½ teaspoon onion powder
½ teaspoon ground fennel
½ teaspoon kosher salt
¼ cup grated Parmesan cheese

Chapter 7

The Importance of Carbohydrates

Carbohydrates are your body's preferred source of energy. They are necessary for healthy function of the brain, central nervous system, muscles, and the metabolism of fat and protein. They include foods that contain sugar, starch, and fiber. When eaten, these foods are broken down into simple sugar molecules for absorption. It is the rate at which these foods break down that determines their nutritive rank.

Simple Carbohydrates

Simple carbohydrates are the sugars. They are grouped by the number of molecules they are made from. Single sugars, or monosaccharides, have one molecule. They include glucose, fructose, and galactose. Sugars that are composed of two molecules are called disaccharides. They include lactose, maltose, sucrose, and honey.

Glucose

Glucose is made by plants during photosynthesis as energy for the plant. Also known as dextrose, it is the human body's first source of energy Most of the carbohydrates you eat are broken down into glucose by the body. It is absorbed directly into the bloodstream, concentrating in the blood. This concentration is measured as your blood sugar level. You must eat 50 to 100 grams of carbohydrates each day to maintain good blood sugar levels. Glucose is found in plants, fruits, and honey.

Fructose and Galactose

Fructose is found in honey, fruits, and plants as well. It is sweeter than glucose and table sugar. Galactose occurs in nature only as one of the two molecules that make up lactose.

Lactose

Also known as milk sugar, lactose is a disaccharide composed of one glucose and one galactose molecule. Found naturally in milk, it is the only carbohydrate that is animal-based. It is not commonly thought of as a sugar because it is not nearly as sweet as glucose.

Maltose

This disaccharide is composed of two glucose molecules. It is mainly seen in sprouting grains and is a vital component of beer. Brewers soak grain, usually barley, in water, until germination. The maltose is also extracted and used to make malt syrup, a common ingredient in artisan breads.

Refined Sugar: Sucrose

Sucrose is ordinary table sugar, derived from sugar cane and sugar beets. It is composed of one glucose and one fructose molecule. It occurs in small amounts in most fruits and is the most widely used sweetener in American homes. Sucrose provides quick energy, but it is stripped of its additional nutrients in the refining process, so it is not the ideal form of carbohydrate. The human body needs the entire natural package of a piece of fruit, or a tablespoon of honey, which, unlike table sugar, also includes fiber, water, vitamins, and minerals. For more on refined sugar, and ways to sweeten your day without it, see Chapter 9.

Honey

This disaccharide is also composed of one glucose and one fructose molecule. Honey is more concentrated than sucrose, which makes it twice as sweet. Consequently, less is needed when it's used as a sweetener. The body breaks down and uses both sucrose and honey in the same way, but honey is a naturally occurring sweetener that needs no refinement. It contains other elements that are considered healthful, including vitamins, minerals, fiber, and antioxidants. Honey can be substituted for granulated sugar as a sweetener, but because it is twice as sweet, use half as much.

Complex Carbohydrates

Complex carbohydrates are found in plant foods that contain starch and fiber. They are known as polysaccharides, meaning more than two sugars. They come in chains of thousands of glucose molecules. In order to be absorbed, your body must break apart these molecule chains. It takes considerably more effort for your body to absorb polysaccharides than it does to absorb single or double sugars.

Starch is found in grains, root vegetables, nuts, seeds, and fruits. It can gelatinize, meaning that it gets thick and absorbs water when heated.

Fiber, mainly found in plant cell walls, comes in two varieties; water-soluble, and water insoluble. Both types of fiber are essential for good health.

Water-soluble fiber includes substances like pectin. When water is added, this fiber absorbs it like a sponge and swells. This type of fiber seems to help lower blood cholesterol levels, especially in conjunction with a diet low in fat. It also tends to delay the emptying of the stomach, so food is absorbed more slowly, causing that full feeling to last longer. Water-soluble fiber is found in beans, some grains, like oats and barley, and fruits and vegetables such as apples and carrots.

Water-insoluble fiber, which includes cellulose, doesn't swell nearly as much. This includes the structural parts of the plant, like skin, seeds, and stems. Bran, and any whole grain that still includes its outer hull, like brown rice, are great sources of insoluble fiber.

Unlike starch, fiber-based polysaccharides cannot be broken apart by our digestive enzymes. It keeps waste moving through the intestines, which helps prevent disorders of the lower intestine. It is thought that these complex carbohydrates may play a role in the prevention of colon cancer by reducing the time cancer-causing agents spend in the intestine.

Refined Flour

White flour is a commonly consumed starch. Made from wheat endosperm, white flour is so refined that it is practically digested before you eat it, and it is converted into sugar as soon as it is consumed.

The refining process strips the grain of both water-soluble and water-insoluble fibers found in its bran and germ. These two nutritious segments of the grain also contain vitamins, proteins, and healthful oils. In whole grains the presence of fiber slows down digestion, and allows time for these important nutrients to be absorbed. Through refinement, many of these nutrients are missing, and digestion and absorption happen quickly, just like simple carbohydrates.

Whole Grains

Whole-grain food products undergo less refinement and still contain healthful fiber. They take longer to digest and allow full absorption of nutrients.

Whole-wheat flour, brown rice, whole-grain pasta, and whole-grain cereals are just some of the foods that are available in most markets. They convert more slowly to sugar, and take longer to be absorbed, making them a healthier choice for your family.

Complex Carbohydrate Recipes

The following recipes are just a sample of the types of dishes that can be made featuring complex carbohydrates. Once you read them, you will no doubt think of similar recipes you and your family will enjoy. Don't hesitate to substitute whole grains in recipes you have historically made with refined ones. And consider adding fresh vegetables and fruits into some of your existing recipes too. It's easier than you think to get your complex carbs!

Carrot Salad

This sweet, crunchy salad is refreshing in the summer, but don't forget about it in the winter. Add pomegranate seeds, dried cranberries, and walnuts for an autumnal touch.

In a large bowl, whisk together oil, vinegar, orange juice, thyme, and salt. Add carrots, raisins, pear, and apple and toss to coat. Chill 1 hour before serving.

SERVES 4

275 calories
8 g fat
56 g carbohydrates
3 g protein
373 mg sodium
7 g fiber

INGREDIENTS
2 tablespoons olive oil
2 tablespoons rice or cider vinegar
¼ cup orange juice
1 tablespoon fresh thyme, minced
½ teaspoon kosher salt
4 cups grated carrots
1 cup raisins
1 pear, diced
1 apple, diced

Homemade Granola

This makes a great trail mix, or it can be stirred into cookie dough, pancake batter, and muffin mix to add healthy crunch and color. And don't forget to use it as a topping for fruit desserts.

1. Preheat oven to 325°F. Coat a baking sheet with pan spray.

2. In a small saucepan, combine oil, honey, and vanilla. Warm it over medium heat until it begins to simmer.

3. Meanwhile, in a large bowl combine oats, flour, bran, germ, and sunflower seeds. Stir in the warm oil mixture and toss together to thoroughly moisten.

4. Spread the granola onto baking sheet in an even, thin layer. Toast in the oven for 1 hour, stirring every 10 minutes to promote even browning.

5. Cool, then mix in raisins, dates, and almonds. Serve with milk or yogurt, or eat it as is for a great snack. Store airtight for up to 1 week at room temperature, or in the refrigerator for up to 1 month.

Ancient Grains
Grains were probably the first foods to be domesticated, and eating them toasted by the handful would have been the easiest way to find nourishment. Romans began flour refinement with millstones as early as 500 B.C.

INGREDIENTS
⅓ cup peanut oil
¼ cup honey
1 teaspoon vanilla extract
4 cups rolled oats
½ cup whole-wheat flour
½ cup oat bran
½ cup wheat germ
*½ cup hulled sunflower
    seeds*
½ cup toasted coconut
½ cup golden raisins
½ cup dried cranberries
1 cup chopped dates
1 cup chopped almonds

Wild Rice with Orange and Almond

The chewy texture of this dish is a nice compliment to the tender flaky meat of sole or halibut.

1. Heat oil in a large sauté pan over high heat. Add leeks and cook until tender. Add wild rice, zest, and almonds and cook 5–10 minutes, stirring, until toasted and brown.

2. Add water and orange juice and bring to a boil. Reduce heat to low, cover, and cook 45–60 minutes, until liquid is absorbed. Add salt and fluff with a fork just before serving. Serve with orange wedges.

This Rice Is Wild

Wild rice comes from a wild marsh grass that is native to the northern United States. It is chewier and nuttier than regular rice, and consequently it is commonly thought to be undercooked.

SERVES 4

378 calories
14 g fat
57 g carbohydrates
10 g protein
305 mg sodium
6 g fiber

INGREDIENTS
2 tablespoons olive oil
2 leeks, chopped thin
1 cup wild rice
Zest of 1 orange
½ cup sliced almonds
1 cup water
2 cups orange juice
½ teaspoon kosher salt
1 orange sliced into wedges

Cracked Wheat Salad

SERVES 6

180 calories
3 g fat
35 g carbohydrates
6 g protein
230 mg sodium
6 g fiber

INGREDIENTS

2 cloves garlic, minced
2 tablespoons fresh oregano, minced
1 teaspoon ground cumin
1 teaspoon ground cinnamon
3 tablespoons olive oil
Juice and zest of 1 lemon
2 cups cooked cracked wheat (follow package directions)
1 head romaine lettuce, shredded
2 cups fresh spinach, shredded
1 red bell pepper, diced
1 cucumber, diced
1 carrot, grated
3 green onions, minced
¼ cup sliced almonds
½ cup golden raisins
½ teaspoon kosher salt

This salad is a meal in itself, but it also makes a stunning side dish. Serve it with turkey or duck, or a nice piece of grilled salmon. It can hold its own next to any assertive flavor.

1. In a large bowl, combine garlic, oregano, cumin, and cinnamon.

2. Whisk in olive oil, lemon juice, and zest.

3. Add wheat, lettuce, spinach, pepper, cucumber, carrot, and onions. Toss and chill 30 minutes. Just before serving, toss in almonds, raisins, and salt.

Fennel and Citrus Salad

This salad is a refreshing mix of flavors and textures. It's perfection on a hot summer day, but make it in the winter too, when interesting citrus fruits are at their peak.

1. In a large bowl, mix together lime juice and zest, honey, salt, black pepper, cayenne pepper, and mint.

2. Drizzle in olive oil while whisking.

3. Add oranges, grapefruit, fennel, and onion and toss to coat.

4. Cover and refrigerate at least 1 hour to allow flavors to mingle.

Fennel

Known as finocchio *in Italian, and sweet anise bulb, this vegetable is native to the Mediterranean and thrives in similar climates. Bulb, leaves, stem, and seed all have a sweet anise scent and flavor. As a vegetable, fennel bulb is delicious grilled, sautéed, braised, or shaved thin, as in this recipe. The seeds turn up whole in tomato sauces, Italian sausages, and rye breads.*

SERVES 4

368 calories
28 g fat
32 g carbohydrates
3 g protein
180 mg sodium
7 g fiber

INGREDIENTS
*Juice and zest of 1 lime
    (about 1 tablespoon of
    juice)
½ teaspoon honey
¼ teaspoon kosher salt
¼ teaspoon ground black
    pepper
¼ teaspoon cayenne pepper
¼ cup chopped fresh mint
½ cup olive oil
3 sweet oranges, peeled,
    sectioned, and diced
1 ruby red grapefruit, peeled,
    sectioned, and diced
1 bulb fennel, shaved thin
1 medium purple onion,
    chopped and soaked in
    cold water for 15–30
    minutes*

Multigrain Crackers

MAKES 15 CRACKERS

121 calories
6 g fat
14 g carbohydrates
3 g protein
115 mg sodium
3 g fiber

INGREDIENTS
⅔ cup warm water
⅓ cup olive oil
½ teaspoon kosher salt
1 teaspoon baking powder
½ cup rolled oats
½ cup buckwheat flour
1–2 cups whole-wheat flour
1 tablespoon sesame seed
1 tablespoon flax seeds
1 tablespoon poppy seeds
1 egg white

The seeds in this recipe are just suggestions. You can experiment with others or keep it simple and pick just one or two.

1. In a large bowl combine water, oil, and salt.

2. Add baking powder, oats, buckwheat flour, and enough whole-wheat flour to create a firm dough.

3. Turn out onto a floured surface and knead for 5 minutes, adding flour only as necessary, until the dough is smooth. Return to the bowl, dust with flour, cover with plastic wrap, and rest at room temperature for 15 minutes.

4. Preheat oven to 425°F. Coat a baking sheet with pan spray.

5. Turn rested dough out onto a floured surface and divide it into three equal portions.

6. Roll each portion to ¼ inch thick with a rolling pin, and pierce each piece all over with a fork.

7. In a small bowl combine sesame, flax, and poppy seeds.

8. Arrange crackers on baking sheet and brush with egg white. Sprinkle with seed mixture and bake until edges are brown, about 10–15 minutes. When cool, break crackers into serving-size pieces.

Easy Rolling

To ease the rolling of this dough, be sure to give it plenty of rest. Gluten proteins tighten whenever a wheat-based dough is worked. Roll it as far as it wants to go, then let it rest and move on to the next piece. After 2–3 minutes, the gluten in the dough will be relaxed and you can roll it much thinner.

Wilted Greens with Garlic

Wilted greens are not meant to be crisp or soggy.
Just slightly limp. Watch the cooking time carefully,
and resist the temptation to overdo it.

1. Heat oil in a large sauté pan over high heat. Add garlic, onions, pecans, and cook until garlic is tender.

2. Add greens, stir, and cover for 1–2 minutes, until wilted but still bright green.

3. Add lemon and salt and stir to coat evenly. Serve immediately, topped with crumbled goat cheese.

Wash It Well

Fresh garden greens need careful cleaning. Most are grown in muddy, sandy soil, and are only lightly cleaned before coming to market. Submerge them in cold water two or three times. Don't worry about drying them. The heat from the sauté pan will evaporate the water away.

SERVES 8

120 calories
11 g fat
5 g carbohydrates
3 g protein
300 mg sodium
2 g fiber

INGREDIENTS
2 tablespoons olive oil
2 cloves garlic, minced
1 cup green onions, chopped
½ cup pecans, chopped
2 cups spinach, cleaned and chopped
2 cups Swiss chard, cleaned and chopped
2 cups beet greens, cleaned and chopped
2 cups turnip greens, cleaned and chopped
Zest and juice of 1 lemon (about 2 tablespoons juice)
½ teaspoon kosher salt
½ cup goat or feta cheese, crumbled

Split Pea Soup

SERVES 6

310 calories
8 g fat
45 g carbohydrates
17 g protein
230 mg sodium
18 g fiber

INGREDIENTS
3 tablespoons olive oil
1 large yellow onion, chopped
2 stalks celery, chopped
1 carrot, chopped
3 cloves garlic, chopped
1 bay leaf
1 teaspoon dried thyme
2 cups split peas, soaked in
    8 cups water overnight,
    then rinsed
Water to cover
½ teaspoon kosher salt
½ teaspoon black pepper

Split peas are legumes, edible seeds inside of a seed pod.
The most common ones are beans and peanuts.
When the seeds are dried, they are called pulses.

1. Heat oil in a large saucepan over high heat. Add onion, celery, carrot and garlic and cook until tender and light brown.

2. Add bay leaf, thyme, and peas; cover with cold water; and bring to a boil.

3. Reduce heat and simmer 1–2 hours, until peas are tender. Season with salt and pepper.

Last-Minute Beans
If you forget the overnight presoak on your beans, here's what to do. Cover the beans with water, bring to a boil for 5 minutes, then remove from heat, cover, and set aside for 1 hour. Cut a bean in half to see if it is fully soaked. If it is, there will be an even color throughout. If not, there will be a dry core.

Sweet Potato Salad

This is an all-American favorite with a healthy twist.
Try serving it warm as a side dish too.

1. Preheat oven to 400°F.

2. Wrap potatoes in foil and bake 1 hour, until tender. Cool completely, then peel and dice.

3. In a large bowl, combine oil, mustard, vinegar, nutmeg, salt, pepper, and rosemary and mix thoroughly.

4. Add potatoes, celery, and onion and toss to coat vegetables evenly with dressing.

5. Chill potato salad for 1 hour before serving. Store refrigerated for 2 days.

A Spud by Any Other Name

Sweet potatoes and yams are very similar, and usually interchangeable. But they are actually from two separate species. Yams are a tuber grown throughout Latin America, Africa, and Asia. They are sweeter and moister than a true sweet potato. A member of the morning glory family, the sweet potato grows in the tropics, is usually yellow, and is much less sweet than the yam. The sweet potato also tends to crumble like a standard baked potato when cooked.

SERVES 4

270 calories
14 g fat
38 g carbohydrates
3 g protein
470 mg sodium
5 g fiber

INGREDIENTS
4 large sweet potatoes or
  yams
¼ cup olive oil
2 tablespoons Dijon mustard
¼ cup cider vinegar
½ teaspoon grated nutmeg
½ teaspoon kosher salt
½ teaspoon ground black
  pepper
1 tablespoon fresh rosemary,
  minced
1 cup celery, chopped
1 medium purple onion,
  chopped and soaked in
  cold water for 15–30
  minutes

Chapter 8

Fats and Oils

The words fat and oil don't really have good connotations. And it's true that too much of these foods can be a very bad thing. However, fat plays a vital role in human health. You need it as part of a healthy diet. You do not, however, need very much. This chapter explains the pros and cons of fats and oils and the right way to include them in your diet.

What Is Fat, and Why Do You Need It?

Fat is necessary but not in the quantities most Americans consume it. You need it to transport fat-soluble vitamins, insulate you in winter, and cushion your falls. For good health, it's important to understand and choose the right kind of fat.

Fat is a macronutrient, providing you with a concentrated source of energy and vital calories. The chemical name for this group of nutrients is *lipids*, and it includes fat, oil, and lecithin. Lipids are found in both plants and animals. In general, when stored at room temperature, fat is solid and oil is liquid.

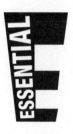

Lecithin is a natural emulsifying agent, which means it can help combine two ingredients that don't naturally combine, such as oil and water. The lecithin in an egg yolk is what lets you emulsify mayonnaise and thick salad dressings. Soy-derived lecithin is used in hundreds of products, including chocolate.

Fatty Acids

Fatty acids are the building blocks of fat. They are linked together in long chains of carbon and hydrogen atoms. If a fatty acid chain is filled to capacity with hydrogen atoms, it is called saturated. This fat is thick, like butter.

If hydrogen is missing, it is called unsaturated. The amount of missing hydrogen determines whether the fat is monounsaturated or polyunsaturated. This type of fat is thin, as in oil.

All fat, including the fat you find in food, is made of a mixture of saturated and unsaturated fats. The majority of the fat a food contains determines its classification as saturated or unsaturated.

Fat is difficult for your body to digest and utilize because fat and water do not mix. Bile is the key to our utilization of fat. Made by the liver and secreted by the gallbladder, bile can break the triglycerides into their components, fatty acids and glycerol, for absorption.

Saturated Fats

This type of fat is found mainly in animal-based foods. It can easily be identified, because the foods are solid at room temperature. You'll find saturated fat in meat, butter, cheese, and lard.

These are the most dangerous types of fat because they appear to raise blood cholesterol levels. They may inhibit the liver's ability to clear out low-density lipoproteins (LDL) and actually stimulate their production. The result is an increased likelihood of atherosclerosis and coronary artery disease.

Saturated fats are found mainly in animals and seldom in plants. The exceptions are palm oil and coconut oil. These plants contain a large amount of saturated fatty acids, which are solid at room temperature. They are free of trans fat, and as such are often encouraged for use in place of hydrogenated oils. Additionally, they are easier for your body to absorb than trans fat.

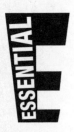

Glycerol is a derivative of carbohydrates that is part of a triglyceride. Separated from the triglyceride it is a clear, sticky, slightly sweet liquid, used as a solvent and emollient in the production of cosmetics and soaps and as a preservative in foods.

Unsaturated Fats

These fats are liquid at room temperature. They are generally referred to as oils, and they come mainly from plant sources. These fats have a shorter shelf life, and are more likely to spoil.

There are two types of unsaturated fats: monounsaturated and polyunsaturated. Monounsaturated fats occur in olive, canola, and nut oils, including peanut oil. Polyunsaturated fats include plant oils like safflower, sunflower, cottonseed, sesame, corn, and soybean. Unsaturated fats have been shown to actually lower the low-density lipoproteins (LDL) in your blood.

The only animal oil that is not saturated is polyunsaturated fish oil. These oils contain healthy omega-3 fatty acids, and are an essential part of a healthy diet. If you do not eat fish at least twice a week, it's a good idea to take fish oil supplements, to ensure you're getting your omega-3s.

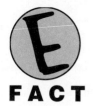

FACT

When fat spoils it is called rancid. Oxygen and light are the main culprits in shortening fat's shelf life. Foods that contain fat should be refrigerated if intended for long-term use.

Trans Fat

This is the worst kind of fat. Trans fat has been shown to both lower the good cholesterol, and raise the bad. Not a healthy prospect. To make matters worse, in recent years trans fats have been used extensively in a manufactured foods.

To make hydrogenated fat, extra hydrogen is added to unsaturated vegetable fat. Trans fats and partially hydrogenated fats are listed on labels.

Since trans fats are artificially saturated, the "E" tails of fatty acids are not straight like natural saturated fats, so they do not line up and pack together tightly. You can see this by comparing the way butter (which has no trans fat) and margarine (which is pure trans fat) spread when chilled.

What Is Cholesterol?

Cholesterol is a type of lipid found in the cells of all body tissues. It is not considered essential because our body makes it in the liver. It is a fatty substance, but unlike fat, it does not provide you with energy. You can't taste it or smell it, but it is in the food you eat, and your body needs it to function properly.

Every cell in your body contains cholesterol. Cholesterol carried in your bloodstream is called blood serum cholesterol. It is transported by blood plasma throughout the body and is used to make cell membranes, bile acids that allow us to digest fats, hormones, and vitamin D. Like so many things, too much cholesterol can be dangerous.

When it is in your food it is called dietary cholesterol. Found mainly in animals, you find lots of it in shrimp, egg yolks, dairy products, and meat.

LDL and HDL

Because fat does not dissolve in water, it is transported through the bloodstream by water-soluble proteins called lipoproteins. They wrap the cholesterol and triglycerides like a package and deliver it throughout the body. From the liver, triglycerides and cholesterol are secreted into plasma, where they are joined with low-density lipoprotein (LDL).

Termed the "bad cholesterol," LDL is thought to increase the risk of heart disease, heart attacks, and stroke. Healthy blood has fairly few large particles of LDL. If too many accumulate, problems occur. When LDL accumulates on the walls of the arteries it can harden them and cause blockage. This is called arterial plaque. If blockage occurs in a main heart artery, a heart attack is the result. If blockage occurs in a major brain artery, stroke can result.

High-density lipoproteins (HDL) circulate in the blood, picking up cholesterol and excess plaque and transporting it back to the liver, where it is excreted as bile. For optimal health, levels of LDL should be low, and levels of HDL should be high. Your cholesterol levels can be determined by a blood test. Healthy ratios of total cholesterol to HDL should be below 5:1, with an optimal ratio of 3.5:1.

Lowering Your Cholesterol Level

Cholesterol is measured in milligrams per deciliter of blood (mg/dl). The numbers for LDL should be low. One hundred and thirty milligrams per deciliter is considered good, 160 is high. If you have heart disease, your target is 70.

HDL levels should be high. In women, the target level range is 50–60 milligrams per deciliter. Men should aim for 40–50. Lower levels are considered risky.

When planning your diet, keep your saturated fat intake low. It should never constitute more than 10 percent of your total fat intake.

Polyunsaturated Fatty Acids: The Omegas

Omega-3 and omega-6 are essential fatty acids, which means you need them for good health, but your body cannot manufacture them. The name of these acids is an indication of where along the fatty acid chain (the "E" tail) hydrogen atoms are missing.

Omega-3 is found in fish oil and plant oils, especially flax. It is believed to reduce inflammation, improve blood circulation, and decrease the thickness of arterial walls, a significant benefit to those with high blood serum cholesterol. Omega-6 is found in nuts, whole grains, legumes, sesame oil, and soy oil. When used together to replace saturated fats, these fatty acids can reduce high blood pressure and cholesterol.

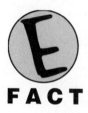

FACT

Flax seeds are primarily used to make linseed oil, but they are also marketed in health food stores. Look for them near the grains, and add them into pilafs, salads, cereals, and breads.

Cooking with Fats

Fats are an important part of cuisine. They carry flavor throughout a recipe, bind and emulsify ingredients, and of course, add flavor. The key to healthy cooking is knowing which fats to use.

Specific Fat Content of Commonly Used Oils

Oil	Saturated Fat	Polyunsaturated Fat	Monounsaturated Fat
Canola Oil	7%	32% (21% omega-6, 11% omega-3)	61%
Coconut Oil	91%	2% (2% omega-6)	7%
Corn Oil	13%	58% (57% omega-6, 1% omega-3)	29%
Flax Seed Oil	9%	73% (16% omega-6, 57% omega-3)	18%

Oil	Saturated Fat	Polyunsaturated Fat	Monounsaturated Fat
Olive Oil	15%	10% (9% omega-6, 1% omega-3)	75%
Safflower Oil	8%	15% (15% omega-6, 1% omega-3)	77%
Sunflower Oil	12%	72% (71% omega-6, 1% omega-3)	16%

Oils

Oil is an essential part of a salad. Without oil, the dressing would slip off the lettuce, and pool at the bottom of the bowl. Just think about the way oil feels when it gets on your hands. Oil spreads flavor throughout a recipe like it spreads on your hands. You need it in recipes, but you don't need that much.

Whenever possible, use mainly monounsaturated oils, which contribute to high-density lipoproteins. Olive and peanut oils are good choices. They have fairly distinctive flavors, and can easily overpower a dish, so use a light hand. If a neutral oil is called for, canola is a good monounsaturated choice.

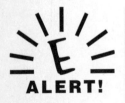

Labels are allowed to read "0 grams" trans fat when there is 0.5 of a gram or less. This means that eating more than one serving can quickly add 1 gram or more of trans fat. It is best to generally limit, if not eliminate, all foods that contain partially hydrogenated oil.

Fats

Like oil, fats are added to recipes to tenderize, moisten, and prolong shelf life. Because they change their consistency when heated, the temperature indicated in the recipe is important.

The most frequent fat used for baking is butter. Unsalted butter is preferred by most bakers and chefs for its superior flavor. The lack of salt gives the cook control over the amount of salt in a recipe. Salted butter can always be detected, as it makes the dish saltier than necessary. If you have no choice but to use salted butter, you should omit the salt from the recipe.

Margarine is never a good choice. Its flavor is inferior, and because it is typically a trans fat, it is an unhealthy food. Also, its higher melting point leaves behind an unpleasant aftertaste. Because vegetable fats do not melt at body temperatures, as animal fats do, margarine coats the tongue, and lingers on the palate long after the food is swallowed.

Butter, although a saturated animal-based fat, is preferable to margarine in maintaining a healthy diet. However, problems occur with any saturated fats when eaten in excess. They are the healthier alternative but should be eaten in moderation, as all fats should be.

Lard is less popular than in the past, but it is often preferred by bakers, especially in pie dough. It creates a superior flakiness that cannot be achieved with butter or shortening, and because it is an animal product, it leaves behind no unpleasant aftertaste. Like butter, lard is preferable to margarine. It is generally rendered from pork, although in other parts of the world it is made from other animal fats too.

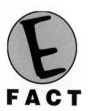

FACT

The USDA suggests that you consume no more than 7 teaspoons of fat and oil each day. This includes not just the added butter on your baked potato, but also the fats and oils found naturally in foods and those added to prepared foods.

Recipes to Replace Traditional Fatty Butters and Oils

The following recipes are flavorful alternatives to fatty bottled dressings, dips, and spreads. Use them for salads and crunchy crudités. Or spread them wherever butter would go, on bread, pasta, and even grilled meats. They are flavorful, nutritious alternatives.

Honey Dijon Vinaigrette

MAKES ABOUT ¾ CUP

970 calories
108 g fat
5 g carbohydrates
0 g protein
1,360 mg sodium
0 g fiber

INGREDIENTS
Juice and zest of 1 lemon
   (about 2 tablespoons)
½ teaspoon kosher salt
½ teaspoon ground black
   pepper
1 tablespoon Dijon mustard
1 tablespoon honey
½ cup olive oil

*Serve this dressing over plain mixed greens, steamed vegetables,
or use it as a marinade for whatever you like to grill.*

In a large bowl, whisk together lemon juice and zest, salt, pepper, mustard, and honey. Slowly drizzle in oil while whisking. Add greens, toss to coat, and serve immediately.

Sesame Rice Vinaigrette

**MAKES ABOUT 1½
CUPS**

1,310 calories
126 g fat
44 g carbohydrates
10 g protein
4,030 mg sodium
2 g fiber

INGREDIENTS
2 cloves garlic, minced
1 tablespoon grated ginger
1 tablespoon black sesame
   seeds
2 tablespoons honey
1 teaspoon grated lemon zest
¼ cup soy sauce
¼ cup rice vinegar
½ cup peanut oil
1 tablespoon sesame oil

*Ginger, garlic, and sesame make a classic trio of Asian flavor. Use
it to marinade chicken, toss into stir-fry, or dress your noodles.*

In a large bowl, combined garlic, ginger, sesame seeds, honey, and lemon zest. Stir in soy sauce and vinegar, slowly drizzle in peanut and sesame oil, then whisk until well combined..

Green Goddess Dressing

This is a lightened version of an old-time favorite. It makes a fresh herby dressing for fresh peas and carrots or a three-bean salad. It's also thick enough to use as a dip, spread onto sandwich bread, or mix into hard boiled eggs for a terrific egg salad.

In a blender or food processor, combine yogurt, oil, onions, and garlic. Pulse the machine to puree. Add tarragon, parsley, thyme, and anchovies, and blend until smooth. Add vinegar slowly, then season with salt and pepper. Chill.

MAKES ABOUT 2 CUPS

1,222 calories
113 g fat
32 g carbohydrates
22 g protein
1,958 mg sodium
5 g fiber

INGREDIENTS
1 cup plain low-fat yogurt
½ cup olive oil
1 bunch scallions
1 clove garlic
½ cup fresh tarragon
½ cup fresh parsley
½ cup fresh thyme
4 anchovy filets
¼ cup tarragon vinegar
½ teaspoon kosher salt
½ teaspoon black pepper

Roasted Garlic Spread

Garlic is an amazing food. Roasted in a hot oven it becomes a sweet, caramelized paste that enhances everything, from bread to pasta, steamed shellfish, or vegetable brochettes. Keep it on hand for when your creativity strikes.

1. Preheat oven to 400°F.

2. Wrap unpeeled garlic bulbs in aluminum foil, and roast 30–60 minutes until soft. Cool completely.

3. Cut garlic bulbs in half and squeeze out soft garlic into a bowl. Add oil, thyme, salt, and pepper and mash with a fork until smooth. Serve warm or cold.

MAKES ABOUT 1 CUP

700 calories
42 g fat
76 g carbohydrates
15 g protein
620 mg sodium
5 g fiber

INGREDIENTS
5 bulbs of garlic
2–4 tablespoons olive oil
1 teaspoon dried thyme
¼ teaspoon kosher salt
¼ teaspoon black pepper

Red Yam Spread

MAKES ABOUT 3 CUPS

510 calories
14 g fat
98 g carbohydrates
8 g protein
1,350 mg sodium
13 g fiber

INGREDIENTS
*1 bulb garlic
2 whole yams or sweet
    potatoes
2 medium carrots
1 tablespoon olive oil
½–¾ cup water
1 tablespoon fresh rosemary,
    minced
½ teaspoon kosher salt
½ teaspoon black pepper
Juice of ½ lemon*

This spread is an excellent substitute for butter or mayonnaise on bread and sandwiches, and it also makes a fantastic dip. Try it with veggies or bread sticks.

1. Preheat oven to 400°F.

2. Wrap unpeeled garlic bulb, yams, and carrots separately in aluminum foil, and roast 30–60 minutes until soft. Cool completely.

3. Cut garlic bulb in half and squeeze out soft garlic into a blender. Peel skin off of yams, and add to blender. Cut carrots into 2-inch chunks and add.

4. Turn on blender and puree, adding oil, then water as needed to create a smooth but thick puree. Add rosemary, salt, pepper, and lemon juice to taste. Chill at least 1 hour, or overnight to allow flavors to mingle.

Tapenade

MAKES ABOUT 2 CUPS

1,212 calories
115 g fat
37 g carbohydrates
13 g protein
9,348 mg sodium
8 g fiber

INGREDIENTS
*4 anchovy filets
1 tablespoon herbes de
    Provence
2 cloves garlic, minced
2 cups kalamata olives, pitted
1 cup capers, drained
½ teaspoon black pepper
Juice and zest of 1 lemon
2 tablespoons olive oil
½ cup Italian parsley*

This tangy spread from the south of France is a Mediterranean classic. Use it as a dip for bread, a marinade, a dressing, or a sauce. Its uses are limited only by your imagination.

1. Combine anchovies, herbes de Provence, and garlic in a blender or food processor and pulse to make a paste.

2. Add olives, capers, pepper, lemon, and olive oil, and blend until smooth.

3. Add parsley last, and pulse briefly to chop and spread throughout. Serve at room temperature.

Use the Good Stuff
Be sure to use kalamata olives, or other similar Greek black olives in brine. The canned black olives you used to stick on your fingertips will not cut it here.

Chapter 9
Sweet, Sweet Sugar

Refined sugar is a major player in our poor national diet. Each American consumes about 150 pounds of it a year. That's nearly 3 pounds a week. Almost a full cup every day. If you think that sounds like a lot, you're right! It's important to make sure you don't consume too much refined sugar and instead get your sweet fix in other, more nutritionally beneficial ways.

How Your Body Uses Sugar

Your body is designed to utilize the sugar in food as energy. Carbohydrates found in natural sugars and starches are broken down into their simple molecular components so they may be absorbed and converted to energy. In addition, these foods have other nutrients that your body needs and uses: vitamins, minerals, proteins, fats, and fiber.

Unfortunately, refined sugar, or sucrose, has no nutritional value. Although it is derived from plants (sugar cane and beets), it has been depleted of all other nutrients. What remains is pure carbohydrate in a form the human body is not built to utilize.

These empty calories (foods that contain calories but no viable nutrition are said to contain "empty calories") cannot all possibly be used and are stored in the liver in the form of glycogen. When the liver is full, excess glycogen is taken to the blood in the form of fatty acids and transported for storage all over the body, but particularly in areas that are relatively inactive, including your belly, butt, breasts, and thighs. When these areas are full, the fatty acids are distributed between your organs, reducing their ability to function.

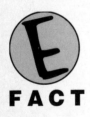

Sugar cane originated in the Pacific Islands, migrated to Asia, the Middle East, and India. Crusaders brought "sweet salt" back from their expeditions, and by the 1400s sugar cane plantations were in full production throughout the Mediterranean. By the 1600s production began in the Caribbean, where it flourished. In the 1700s beets became a popular sugar source when a British blockade denied Napoleon his Caribbean imports.

Your body reacts so strongly to a sudden influx of pure carbohydrate that you can physically feel a rush of energy. Unlike the sugar you get from fruits, milk, or honey, refined sugar is metabolized instantly. And once your body uses it, it craves more, and sends you into withdrawal. If more is not consumed, you experience the inevitable crash. Your body reacts to what is essentially poison by sending nutrients to help keep you in balance. Vitamins, minerals, and enzymes rush to the rescue, resulting in depletion of these nutrients throughout the body.

Sure, carbohydrates are essential for good nutrition. But you were never meant to eat it in a refined state. Your body needs the full benefit of the nutrients that come with a piece of fruit or even a taste of honey. These natural foods take time to digest, entering the body slowly, and are put to use where and when they are needed.

Curbing Your Sugar Intake

Human babies respond to sugar quite early. The taste is innately pleasant because the calorie-rich carbohydrates are an essential energy source for humans. The taste for all things sweet develops as you age, but society has helped it along. In the twentieth century the demand for sugar skyrocketed. Americans went from an annual consumption of a mere 5 pounds in the 1890s to the current intake of 150 pounds. How is this possible?

Soda pop is a major contributor to our immense sugar intake. This is not a beverage that is designed to quench your thirst. It is nothing more than liquid candy. But many Americans consume it with every meal. Kids can even buy it at school.

Sugar absorbs water. In baking, this phenomenon helps keep products moist. In your body it just makes you thirsty. As a result, drinking beverages with sugar to quench your thirst is counterproductive. This, coupled with the craving for sugar that comes after sugar is consumed, equals a guaranteed repeat customer for the soda pop company.

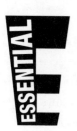

Cats, from large jungle cats down to domestic house cats, are unable to recognize sweetness. In the wild, they're strictly meat eaters, so they have evolved without the sweet taste receptor. You can test it by offering your pets a bowl of water and a bowl of sugar water. Dogs will feed their sweet teeth.

The other contributor to America's enormous sugar consumption is hidden sugar. It is in almost everything you eat. Sure, you know it's in the obvious stuff, like soda and cookies and candy. But it's also in ketchup, mayonnaise, salad dressings, fruit juice, bread, cereal, soups, pizza, pasta, yogurt, and cheese. And when foods are marketed as fat free, there's a good possibility the sugar is increased to raise palatability.

Check the labels of the food in your cupboard, and unless it is specifically a sugar-free product, chances are it will have sugar in it. But be sure to look carefully. Sugar has other names, including dextrose, glucose, fructose, lactose, corn syrup, sorghum, galactose, invert sugar, and malt or maltose.

Refined Versus Natural Sugar

You cannot escape all the sugar in foods, nor should you. You need it for survival, and let's not forget that sugar is yummy. But there are some sugars that are better than others. There are ways to get the sugar you need, eliminate what you don't, and still have a pleasurable life.

Granulated Sugar

Commonly referred to as white sugar or table sugar, it is made both from sugar cane and sugar beets. They are generally interchangeable, although cane sugar is preferable for candy work, as it tends to crystallize less than beet sugar.

Brown Sugar

This is white sugar that has molasses added to it, although traditionally brown sugar was less refined. The manufacturing process makes it more economically feasible to refine it all, then add molasses, removed during refinement, back in. Light brown sugar has less molasses, and less flavor, than dark brown. They are interchangeable, and their use should be determined by your taste preferences.

Molasses

This is the by-product of the sugar refinement process. Molasses is widely used for its flavor and color. Unsulfured is considered the finest quality, and is made by boiling ripened sugar cane. Sulfured molasses is made from green sugar cane that is treated with sulfur dioxide during extraction, which acts as a preservative. Blackstrap molasses is made from subsequent boiling, and while it has less sugar, it contains large amounts of micronutrients, including iron, calcium, magnesium, and potassium. It is commonly used as a diet supplement, as well as in cattle feed and large-scale food manufacturing. Molasses from sugar beets is a different product and is not marketed to the general public.

Corn Syrup

This sweet syrup is made from corn starch. Similar to the way carbohydrates are broken down in your system, acids and enzymes are added to liquefied corn starch, turning it into glucose with a small amount of dextrose and maltose. Another enzyme is used to create high-fructose corn syrup. It is a complicated process, but even with such a big production it is cheaper to produce and transport than sugar. High-fructose corn syrup has the same level of sweetness as sugar, and because it is less expensive, it is used far more frequently in manufacturing. In fact, Americans now consume more high-fructose corn syrup than any other form of sugar.

Honey

In an effort to curb your intake of refined sugars, think about using honey as a sweetener. Twice as sweet as sucrose, honey has a unique flavor that enhances baked goods. It is rich in antioxidants, and long-term use has been shown to provide health benefits, including improved digestion, a stronger immune system, and lower cholesterol.

Date Sugar

Date sugar is another option. It is nothing but ground dried dates, but it is equally as sweet as refined sugar. It has the added benefits of fiber, which slows down its absorption into your body, and all the vitamins and minerals of dates. It does not melt like sugar, so it's not good for coffee. But it is terrific in cakes, and wherever you shake sugar for sweet crunchy toppings.

Maple Syrup

The majority of syrups in your market are made from corn syrup. But the real thing, made from reduced maple sap, is full of minerals and antioxidants. Lighter colored maple syrup is less concentrated than the dark stuff.

Unrefined Dehydrated Cane Sugar

This is sugar from sugar cane, but it has been extracted naturally, retaining all of its vitamins and minerals. The glycemic index (GI) measures how quickly food raises your blood sugar. Glucose, one of the fastest carbohydrates, has a GI of 100. High numbers are good for quickly raising blood sugar and for quick bursts of intense exercise. Low GI numbers are best for general activities or long periods of steady exertion.

Agave Nectar

From the same plant that gives us tequila comes a syrup sweeter than cane sugar but with a very low glycemic index, so it is absorbed more slowly into the bloodstream. This prevents it from raising blood sugar levels significantly, eliminating the highs and lows associated with sugar intake. For this reason, it's favored among those with diabetes and hypoglycemia. Creative chefs use agave nectar anywhere sugar or honey will go: barbeque sauces, marinades, baked goods, etc. It adds a distinctive sweet flavor, reminiscent of tequila. Agave nectar is available through Internet sources (*www.rawagave. com, www.agavenectar.com*) and at health food stores.

Stevia

This sweetener is extracted from an herb (called stevia, sweetleaf, or sugarleaf) that is 300 times sweeter than granulated sugar but with a gylcemic index of zero. This means it will not affect your blood sugar level, giving you no highs or lows. It doesn't melt, or caramelize like sugar, but it dissolves nicely in liquids.

Sugar Myths

Because sugar is such a beloved part of the American diet, it is no surprise that there are a few old wives' tales that have sprung up around it.

Myth 1: Sugar Makes You Fat

The fact is that sugar is a part of a natural, healthy diet, and consumed as part of a well-balanced, natural diet, it will not cause excessive weight gain. Unfortunately, a well-balanced natural diet is not what most Americans consume. Most Americans eat a hefty amount of foods that contain added sugar. Added sugar is found in nearly all manufactured foods, including soda, juice, breads, condiments, cereals, and yogurts. These added sugars are considered the main contributor to the rise of obesity in America.

Myth 2: Sugar Is Addicting

Human DNA has a built-in craving for sweet food, but not for refined sugar. Primitive peoples needed to pad their bodies with excess weight for the long winter and against famine, but they relied on sweet foods that were nutritious and nontoxic. We no longer have such needs, but we still experience the physiological desire for sweets. The key to combating this cruel side of Mother Nature is to exercise some restraint. Get your sweet fix in as natural a form as you can and eat only enough to initially satisfy that sweet tooth.

Myth 3: A Healthy Diet Eliminates All Sugar

It would be unhealthy, and practically impossible, to eliminate all sugar from a healthy diet. Sugar is a natural element in every kind of food, except meat. But eliminating the added sugars that do not naturally occur in foods is a great way to increase the nutritive values of your daily diet. Check labels regularly and opt for homemade over packaged foods to get a handle on your sugar intake.

Myth 4: White Sugar Is the Worst

While it is true that white refined sugar is bad, it is no worse than brown sugar, "raw" sugar, powdered sugar, corn syrup, or any of the ingredients on your food labels that end in "-ose." All refined sugars should be limited in favor of natural sugars. It is true that natural sugars break down in the same way as refined sugars, but it takes longer, and they provide additional nutrients.

Artificial Sweeteners

Also called nonnutritive sweeteners, there are five products that the Food and Drug Administration (FDA) has approved for human consumption. Testing is ongoing with all of these products, so health and safety is still in question.

Saccharine

Used as an artificial sweetener for more than 100 years, saccharine is over 200 times sweeter than sucrose, and it doesn't raise blood sugar levels. But in the 1970s it was found to cause cancer in rats and a ban was proposed. Because the effect has not been seen in humans, the product is still in use, but the labels must carry a warning. Saccharine is found in Sweet'N Low, Sweet Twin, and Necta Sweet.

Aspartame

This artificial sweetener is used in thousands of products all over the world. It has calories (4 calories per gram), but it is about 200 times sweeter than sucrose, so you don't need much. A can of diet soda typically contains about 225 mg. There are many claims of adverse health effects from the ingestion of aspartame, including headaches, dizziness, anxiety, cramps, multiple sclerosis, lupus, and cancer. Headaches and depression have indeed been shown to occur in people with sensitivities who ingest aspartame. Aspartame isn't safe for people with a rare hereditary disease called phenylketonuria (PKU), and this is indicated on the label. Brain tumors have resulted in rats, but studies continue on the correlation between aspartame and human cancer. Dieters have also reported that aspartame increases appetite. Aspartame is found in NutraSweet and Equal.

Acesulfame Potassium K

Two hundred times sweeter than sucrose, this product is generally used as a flavor enhancer and preservative. It contains the carcinogen methylene chloride, which, with long exposure, causes headaches, nausea, depression, liver and kidney disease, and cancer in humans. There has been only initial testing. Acesulfame potassium K is found in Sunett and Sweet One.

Sucralose

This sweetener is 600 times sweeter than sucrose. It is the most recent addition to the list of artificial sweeteners and is currently used in nearly 5,000 products. Its big draw is that it can be used in baking, which other artificial sweeteners cannot. It has calories (391 calories per 110 grams), but because so little is needed, the amounts are small per serving and do not need to be reported on labels. The product is said to be made from sugar, but that is a bit misleading. Reports indicate it was discovered when scientists were treating sugar with a multitude of chemicals trying to create an insecticide. Adverse symptoms from sucralose consumption include gastrointestinal disorders, skin irritation, chest pain, anxiety, and depression. Sucralose is found in Splenda.

Neotame

This is a new sweeter version of aspartame, more than 7,000 times sweeter than sucrose. It was developed to be a version of aspartame safe for people with PKU. The FDA has given initial approval, but study continues. Neotame is used widely in food manufacturing.

Sweet Tooth–Soothing Sugar-Substitute Recipes

The following recipes were developed using natural sucrose replacements. Don't forget to use these replacements in other recipes, too.

Chocolate Brownies

SERVES 6–8

470 calories
32 g fat
44 g carbohydrates
9 g protein
280 mg sodium
6 g fiber

INGREDIENTS
¾ cup canola oil
1½ cups date sugar
½ cup water
3 eggs
¾ cup whole-wheat flour
½ cup cocoa powder
¾ teaspoon baking powder
½ teaspoon kosher salt
½ cup chopped walnuts
½ cup carob chips

One of these brownies and a tall glass of milk can make even homework seem fun.

1. Preheat oven to 350°F.

2. Coat a 9" × 13" brownie pan with pan spray.

3. In a large bowl combine oil, sugar, water, and eggs and whip together until frothy.

4. Sift in flour, cocoa powder, and baking powder.

5. Add salt and stir until well blended. Fold in walnuts and carob chips.

6. Transfer to prepared pan and bake for 20–25 minutes, until firm. Cool completely before serving.

Apple Butter

MAKES ABOUT
2 CUPS

1,990 calories
0 g fat
543 g carbohydrates
1 g protein
310 mg sodium
62 g fiber

INGREDIENTS
4 pounds apples, mixed
    varieties
1 cup water
1 cup honey
Pinch salt
1 cinnamon stick
1 clove
1 tablespoon cider vinegar

If you've never had apple butter you're in for a treat. It is essentially an apple jam, but it has been cooked to a deep caramel flavor and color. Use it as you would use jam, on bread, pancakes, or wherever you prefer.

1. Peel and core apples, and chop them into medium-size pieces.

2. Combine apples in a large pot with water and cook over high heat until soft, stirring occasionally.

3. When apples are soft, add honey, salt, cinnamon, clove, and vinegar.

4. Continue cooking, stirring frequently to prevent scorching, until the water has evaporated and the apples are thick. A spoonful should maintain its rounded shape. Cool completely and refrigerate.

Chocolate Cake

This is a lovely, moist cake that is great on its own, but even better smothered with fresh berries.

1. Preheat oven to 350°F.

2. Coat a 9" × 13" rectangular pan with pan spray.

3. In a large bowl, stir together flour, date sugar, cocoa, baking soda, and salt.

4. In a separate bowl combine water, oil, vinegar, and vanilla.

5. Slowly stir the oil mixture into the flour mixture.

6. Pour into prepared pan and bake for 20–25 minutes, until a toothpick inserted at the center of the cake comes out clean. Cool completely.

SERVES 6–8

280 calories
15 g fat
35 g carbohydrates
5 g protein
300 mg sodium
3 g fiber

INGREDIENTS
*1⅔ cups unbleached white flour
¾ cup date sugar
¼ cup cocoa powder
1 teaspoon baking soda
½ teaspoon kosher salt
1 cup water
½ cup canola oil
1 teaspoon cider vinegar
1 teaspoon vanilla*

Carrot Cake

The pineapple and nuts are traditional add-ins, but they are just suggestions. You can add any other garnish to this batter, including raisins, candied ginger, or fresh berries.

1. Preheat oven to 350°F. Coat a 9" × 13" rectangular pan with pan spray.

2. Sift together flour, baking powder, baking soda, salt, spices, and sugar and set aside.

3. In a large bowl, mix together oil, eggs, carrots, and pineapple. Slowly add the sifted ingredients, combine thoroughly, and fold in half the nuts.

4. Pour into prepared pan and bake for 30–45 minutes, until a toothpick inserted at the center of the cake comes out clean. Cool completely.

5. For the frosting, beat the cream cheese, vanilla, and honey together until smooth and creamy. Spread on top of cooled carrot cake, and sprinkle with remaining nuts. To serve, slice into squares.

SERVES 10

700 calories
47 g fat
65 g carbohydrates
10 g protein
650 mg sodium
5 g fiber

INGREDIENTS:
*2 cups all-purpose flour
2 teaspoons baking powder
1½ teaspoons baking soda
1 teaspoon salt
2 teaspoons cinnamon
2 teaspoons nutmeg
½ teaspoon clove
2 cups date sugar
1½ cups vegetable oil
4 eggs
2 cups grated carrot
1 cup chopped pineapple
1 cup chopped walnuts, divided
1 (8-ounce) package light cream
    cheese, softened
1 tablespoon vanilla
½ cup honey*

Banana Walnut Bread

SERVES 8

380 calories
22 g fat
43 g carbohydrates
8 g protein
350 mg sodium
7 g fiber

INGREDIENTS
1¾ cups whole-wheat flour
½ teaspoon kosher salt
1 tablespoon baking powder
1 cup walnuts, chopped
⅓ cup peanut oil
⅔ cup date sugar
1 teaspoon grated orange
   zest
2 eggs
1½ cups ripe banana pulp
½ cup shredded coconut

This classic bread is great for breakfast, but you haven't lived until you use it to make a peanut butter sandwich.

1. Preheat oven to 350°F.

2. Coat a loaf pan with pan spray, and line with a strip of parchment or wax paper.

3. Sift together the flour, salt, and baking powder. Stir in walnuts and set aside.

4. Beat together oil, date sugar, and zest until creamy.

5. Add the eggs 1 at a time to the sugar mixture and mix.

6. Stir in bananas.

7. Slowly stir in the premixed dry ingredients until smooth.

8. Fill loaf pan to ½ inch from the top and sprinkle with coconut.

9. Bake until risen, firm, and golden brown, about 50 minutes. A toothpick inserted into the middle should come out clean. Cool for 15 minutes before removing from pan.

Homemade Berry Jam

This jam can easily be made with peaches, apricots, cherries, or plums. Try adding a cinnamon stick, vanilla bean, or bay leaf for an interesting added layer of flavor.

1. In a large sauté pan, combine berries, honey, lemon juice and zest, and salt.

2. Place over high heat, and stir, mashing berries, until the juice begins to run.

3. Reduce heat, and continue to cook, stirring occasionally, until the berries are swimming in juice.

4. Continue to cook and stir until the liquid is evaporated and the jam is thick.

5. Taste and adjust seasoning with honey or lemon juice as needed. Cool completely and refrigerate.

How Sweet It Is

This recipe calls for honey as needed. That's because fruit never tastes the same way twice. Seasons, varieties, soil, growers, and storage all play a role in the level of sweetness, acidity, and overall flavor. So use your taste buds and adjust accordingly.

MAKES ABOUT 2 CUPS

520 calories
3 g fat
131 g carbohydrates
6 g protein
300 mg sodium
32 g fiber

INGREDIENTS
4 cups raspberries or blackberries
¼ cup honey, and more as needed
Juice and zest of ½ lemon
Pinch kosher salt

Carob Chip Oatmeal Cookies

**MAKES ABOUT
2 DOZEN COOKIES**

per cookie
210 calories
11 g fat
25 g carbohydrates
4 g protein
120 mg sodium
2 g fiber

INGREDIENTS
1½ cups rolled oats
1½ cups whole-wheat flour
½ cup date sugar
1 teaspoon baking powder
1 teaspoon baking soda
1 teaspoon nutmeg
1 egg
½ cup honey
½ cup peanut oil
⅔ cup nonfat milk
*1 cup unsweetened carob
    chips*
1 cup pecans, chopped

*These cookies make a great snack. They are full of whole grains,
fiber, protein, and iron. Also, they're so yummy!*

1. Preheat oven to 350°F.

2. Line a baking sheet with parchment paper.

3. In a large bowl, stir together oats, flour, date sugar, baking powder, baking soda, and nutmeg.

4. In a separate bowl, whisk together egg, honey, oil, and milk, then add to dry ingredients. Mix thoroughly, then fold in carob and nuts.

5. Drop dough by the heaping tablespoonful on prepared pan, two inches apart.

6. With moistened fingers or the bottom of a glass dipped in water, press the dough flat.

7. Bake 10 minutes, until golden brown. Cool completely.

Carob
*Carob chips are made from the dried ground pods of the evergreen
carob tree. These pods have a subtle natural sweetness, and a flavor
similar to chocolate. Unsweetened carob chips are available in health
food stores, and on the Internet.*

Date Sugar Cookies

These chewy cookie nuggets will satisfy any sugar craving.

1. Preheat oven to 350°F. Line a baking sheet with parchment paper.

2. In a large bowl stir together dates, pecans, coconut, date sugar, and egg. Mix well.

3. Roll this mixture into walnut-sized balls and place on prepared baking sheet, one inch apart.

4. Bake for 10–15 minutes, until golden brown. Cool before serving.

MAKES 2 DOZEN COOKIES

per cookie
80 calories
4 g fat
10 g carbohydrates
1 g protein
15 mg sodium
1 g fiber

INGREDIENTS

1 cup chopped dates
1 cup chopped pecans
1 cup unsweetened shredded coconut, divided
¾ cup date sugar
1 egg
Pinch kosher salt

Homemade Coconut Ice Cream

SERVES 6

642 calories
53 g fat
37 g carbohydrates
10 g protein
270 mg sodium
6 g fiber

INGREDIENTS
3–4 cups of ice
3 cups half-and-half
1 (15-ounce) can coconut
   milk
8 egg yolks
½ cup agave syrup
4 cups coconut, unsweetened
   shredded, or fresh grated
1 tablespoon coconut extract
½ teaspoon kosher salt

Coconuts have saturated fat, but it is more easily absorbed by our bodies than animal fat. In the coconut milk can, the fat rises to the surface as it sits on the shelf. Be sure to shake up the can before you open it.

1. Fill a large bowl with ice, and then set another large bowl on top of the ice. Have a strainer nearby, and set all this aside.

2. Bring the half-and-half and coconut milk to a boil in a large saucepan.

3. In a small bowl, whisk together agave syrup and egg yolks.

4. When milk mixture is at the boil, temper ½ cup of this mixture into the yolks and whisk quickly to combine.

5. Pour the warmed yolks back into the saucepan and, over high heat, whisk immediately and vigorously until the mixture begins to resemble thick cream, about 2 minutes. Strain immediately into the bowl sitting on ice. Stir periodically until cool.

6. Meanwhile, toast shredded coconut. Spread it in a thin layer on a baking sheet and bake in a 350°F oven, stirring every 5 minutes, until the color is dark brown and even, about 20 minutes.

7. Add hot toasted coconut to the cooling custard, stir, and steep until cool.

8. When the custard is completely cool, strain out the shredded coconut, squeezing out every last bit.

9. Stir in the extract and salt, then run through an ice cream machine, according to manufacturer's instructions. Freeze the ice cream for several hours for firm scoops.

Fat Content
Lower fat content by using skim milk and egg whites. Use 3 cups of skim milk, and 8 egg whites. The result is not as rich, but it is certainly refreshing.

Chapter 10

Fiber

Fiber is a term used for several plant materials that your body can't digest. It is a polysaccharide (multiple molecule sugar) carbohydrate, but unlike starch and sugar, fiber cannot be broken apart by your digestive enzymes. A healthy diet needs a variety of fiber sources. Fiber promotes a healthy digestive system, and can reduce cholesterol levels. Healthy daily fiber intake for a 2,000-calorie-a-day diet should average about thirty grams. Unfortunately, most Americans get only half of what they need.

Soluble and Insoluble Fiber

There are two kinds of fibers, water-soluble and water-insoluble. Both are necessary for good health. Water-soluble fibers have been shown to help lower blood cholesterol levels when included in a low-fat diet. Low-density lipoprotein (LDL) cholesterol levels appear to drop more than with a low-fat diet alone. In addition, these fibers slow the rate of digestion, which in turn increases the rate of absorption. The longer a food is in the intestines, the more nutrients can be absorbed from it. Oats have the most soluble fiber of any grain, followed by barley and brown rice. Soluble-fiber can also be found in legumes, citrus, berries, and apples.

Insoluble fiber, such as cellulose, comes from the skin, stems, and seeds of plants. It is linked to lowered risk and slower progression of cardiovascular disease. And because it keeps waste moving through the intestines, it may help prevent colon cancer by reducing the time cancer-causing agents are in the intestine. Fiber swells up as it absorbs water, which delays the emptying of the stomach. Not only is this good for absorption, but it makes you feel full longer. The extra chewing it takes slows down your meal too, which gives your stomach time to tell your brain it's full.

Bran and any whole-grain food that still includes its outer hull, such as brown rice, are good sources of insoluble fiber. Nuts, fruit in its skin, and vegetables, including cabbage, celery, carrots, beets, and cauliflower, are also excellent sources.

Daily Requirements

The average adult needs about three cups of vegetables and four to five cups of grains every day. Most Americans get nowhere near that amount. As a general rule, one-third of your plate at every meal should be filled with fiber-rich grains, and every snack should include either fiber-filled fruit, vegetables, or grains.

As a country, we eat only 10 percent of the amount of fiber we ate at the turn of the twentieth century. Americans eat a lot of wheat, but it is made into highly refined flour and mixed with refined sugars and hydrogenated oils until it is no longer recognizable (by your body) as grain. Refined grains are partially responsible for the epidemic of weight gain, type II diabetes, and cardiovascular disease. In addition, lack of fiber in the modern diet seems to be linked to gastrointestinal disorders, including several forms of cancer.

Increased intake of fiber can reduce these risks dramatically. As an added bonus, fiber sources also contain, vitamins, minerals, protein, and only limited oils.

Fiber Supplements

Fiber supplements are often prescribed for constipation and other bowel disorders. But these prescriptions are generally meant to be used for a limited time, until the conditions are alleviated. Lack of exercise, insufficient fluid intake, and a general lack of fiber intake all contribute to these malfunctions, as do some medications and surgical procedures.

It's easy to get too much fiber with supplements. This is problematic, as fiber binds to some minerals, including calcium and iron, preventing absorption. The conclusion is that fiber is best taken naturally. It's not that hard to get the fiber that you need. Look for bread that has at least two grams of fiber per slice. Have high-fiber snacks like popcorn and fresh veggies. Add berries and dried fruit to high-fiber cereal for breakfast. By getting your fiber this way, you also get all the other nutrients associated with those foods, which you need every day anyway.

Natural Sources of Fiber

Following is a list that includes some common grains that can be used to make pilafs similar to those in this chapter's recipes. They are not difficult to cook, and they offer much more in the way of flavor than refined plain white rice. The basic method of cooking grain is to boil it in water. The ratio of water to grain varies, but it is generally two and a half to three parts water to one part grain. Water is boiled, then the grains are added and simmered over low heat with the lid on to trap the steam. This tenderizes the grain by encouraging absorption of water. It is also possible to cook grain as you would pasta, in a large pot of boiling water, straining out the grain when tender. This method loses some nutrients, but it is convenient if the optimal water-to-grain ratio is unknown.

While simply boiling grains works to cook them, their flavor is greatly enhanced by toasting. Several recipes in this chapter use a small amount of oil to toast the grain until brown and fragrant, giving it a nutty, rich flavor.

- **Amaranth:** This tiny grain, grown at high altitude, originated in the Andes and Himalayas. It is commonly popped like popcorn, and bound together with honey, like an ancient Rice Krispies treat.
- **Barley:** This grain is less popular than it used to be. It is rarely seen outside of soup, but it can make delicious side dishes and casseroles. Pearled or polished barley has the bran removed. Hulled barley has the bran intact and is the more healthful choice.
- **Buckwheat:** This is not really a grain but the seed of an herb native to Russia. It is commonly ground into flour and used in a variety of breads. It is also known as kasha, which is a toasted buckwheat groat that is cooked like rice.
- **Bulgur:** These wheat kernels have been steamed, dried, and crushed. They do not require cooking but need only be soaked in cold water. Bulgur is the base of Middle Eastern tabouli salad.
- **Couscous:** This is not a grain, but a coarse granular semolina, which is a flour made from protein-rich wheat called durum. Couscous cooks quickly, and is a terrific vehicle for more flavorful sauces and stews. It is most associated with the cuisine of Morocco.
- **Cracked Wheat:** This wheat is crushed with the bran intact. It is not pre-steamed like bulgur, so it must be cooked in boiling water like rice.
- **Kamut:** This is an ancient strain of wheat, more than twice the size of modern wheat kernels, with a greater amount of protein. It can be made into pilafs, kneaded into breads, or ground into flour.
- **Millet:** Used mostly as bird seed in the United States, this small grain is a staple food in much of the world, due to its high protein content and pleasantly mild flavor. It cooks up soft and delicate, absorbing flavors.
- **Oats:** Most Americans eat oatmeal from rolled, quick-cooking oats. But oats are also available steel cut, as groats (grains that are hulled and crushed) or as flour.
- **Quinoa:** This tiny grain has gained recent popularity, but it is actually an ancient food consumed by the Incas and Aztecs. It is extremely high in protein and easy to cook, and it has a pleasant crunch.

- **Rye:** Closely related to barley and wheat, it is available rolled like oats or as rye berries, in which the grain is whole with the bran removed. Rye flour is commonly used in bread making, although it contains no gluten.
- **Spelt:** This is an ancient relative of wheat, native to southern Europe. Spelt has more protein than common wheat and, like Kamut, has huge nutty grains.
- **Teff:** A tiny grain from Africa, teff is high in protein, calcium, and iron. It is eaten as porridge or ground into flour and used to make the Ethiopian bread injera.
- **Triticale:** This is a nutritious hybrid of wheat and rye, available in whole grain of flour forms.
- **Wheat Berries:** These are whole grains of wheat stripped of their outer hulls.

Fruit and Vegetable Fiber

The more skins and seeds you eat with your fruits and veggies, the more fiber you'll be getting. Some great sources are those that are mostly skin and seeds, like raspberries, blackberries, corn, kiwi, cucumbers, figs, and dried fruits. Stems are good too, and while you may not relish the thought of eating a stem, consider that celery and asparagus are nothing but stem.

All the green leafy vegetables are loaded with fiber. You can see it in the veins of the leaves. Artichokes, brussels sprouts, green beans, and onions are all good sources too. And the sweet potato is a fiber gold mine.

Keep plenty of these fiber-rich fruits and vegetables on hand. Keeping them washed and cut into serving sizes will encourage healthy snacking. Make fresh salads part of everyday eating, and use fresh and dried fruits to combat a sweet tooth.

Fiber-Rich Recipes

The recipes in this chapter are designed to help you meet your daily recommended fiber intake. Men should aim for thirty-eight grams of fiber, and women need at least twenty-five grams of dietary fiber every day.

Mixed-Grain Pilaf

SERVES 4–6

200 calories
8 g fat
27 g carbohydrates
6 g protein
410 mg sodium
5 g fiber

INGREDIENTS

3 tablespoons olive oil
1 large yellow onion, chopped
1 carrot, chopped
1 stalk celery, chopped
3 cloves garlic, minced
1 tablespoon sesame seeds
¼ cup wild rice
¼ cup barley
½ teaspoon kosher salt
3 cups chicken broth
¼ cup brown rice
¼ cup cracked wheat
2 cups asparagus or green beans, cut in 1-inch pieces

*Timing is the key to this recipe, because
each grain absorbs liquid at a different rate.*

1. Heat oil in a large sauté pan over high heat.

2. Add onions, carrots, celery, and garlic and cook until tender.

3. Add sesame seeds, wild rice, and barley and cook 5–10 minutes, stirring, until toasted and brown.

4. Add salt and broth, and bring to a boil. Reduce heat to low, cover, and cook 15 minutes.

5. At the 15-minute mark, stir in brown rice and cook another 15 minutes.

6. Add the cracked wheat and cook 10 minutes.

7. Add asparagus or beans and cook a final 5 minutes, until water is absorbed and beans are bright green.

8. Fluff with a fork just before serving, and top with sliced almonds.

Be Creative

Some of the more obscure grains listed earlier in the chapter would work well in this dish. They all require a different water-to-grain ratio, so check the package.

Multigrain Bread

This bread is great for sandwiches, or form it into dinner rolls. These specialty grains are available at any health food store, and can be ordered online.

1. In a medium bowl, combine water, cracked wheat, yeast, and honey and let stand 30 minutes.

2. Add rye flour, oats, corn meal, whole-wheat flour, and salt and combine thoroughly.

3. Add enough bread flour to create a firm dough.

4. Turn dough out onto a floured surface and knead, adding flour only when necessary, until it becomes smooth and elastic, about 8–10 minutes.

5. Return to the bowl, cover with plastic wrap, and set in a warm place to rise until doubled in volume, about 1 hour.

6. Coat 2 loaf pans with pan spray and line with a strip of parchment or wax paper.

7. Turn dough out onto a floured surface and, with a rolling pin, roll into a 18" × 24" rectangle. Starting on a long edge, roll the dough up into a log. Cut the log into two (9-inch) loaves and place each loaf in a pan, seam side down. Dust with flour, cover with plastic wrap, and let rise again for 30 minutes.

8. Preheat oven to 350°F.

9. Combine egg with 1 tablespoon of water and brush over the surface of the breads.

10. Bake until golden brown and firm, about 50–60 minutes. Cool completely before slicing. Store bread for 2 days at room temperature wrapped airtight, or freeze for up to 2 weeks.

Freshness First
Store unused grains in the freezer for up to 4 months to ensure freshness.

MAKES 2 LOAVES

per loaf
1,530 calories
14 g fat
318 g carbohydrates
52 g protein
1,210 mg sodium
22 g fiber

INGREDIENTS
2½ cups warm water
¼ cup cracked wheat
2 (.25-ounce) packages active dry yeast
½ cup honey
¼ cup rye flour
¼ cup rolled oats
¼ cup corn meal
1 cup whole-wheat flour
1 teaspoon kosher salt
3–4 cups bread flour
1 egg
2 tablespoons hulled sunflower seeds
2 tablespoons sesame seeds

Five-Bean Succotash

SERVES 4

460 calories
9 g fat
79 g carbohydrates
22 g protein
1,280 mg sodium
19 g fiber

INGREDIENTS
2 tablespoons olive oil
1 small yellow onion,
    chopped
1 cup corn kernels, fresh or
    frozen
1 cup lima beans, fresh or
    frozen
1 (15-ounce) can black beans,
    rinsed
1 cup green beans, fresh or
    frozen
1 (15-ounce) can chickpeas,
    rinsed
1 (15-ounce) can kidney
    beans, rinsed
½ teaspoon kosher salt
2 tablespoons dried thyme
2 tablespoons chopped fresh
    parsley

The name succotash *comes from the Algonquin word* msickquatash, *meaning "boiled corn or kernels". The colonists probably didn't know this dish, as lima beans didn't arrive until trade routes brought lima beans from Central America.*

1. Heat oil in a large sauté pan over high heat.

2. Add onion and cook until tender.

3. Add corn, lima beans, black beans, green beans, kidney beans, chickpeas, salt, and thyme and cook to warm through.

4. Remove from heat, stir in parsley, and serve.

Sodium Safety
Canned vegetables have added sodium as a preservative. Choose low-sodium varieties if you can, and be sure to rinse them thoroughly.

Brown Rice Pilaf with Apricots

The key to this simple dish is toasting the grain in oil before the liquid is added, which gives it a rich nutty flavor. This dish can also be cooked in the oven. After you bring the liquid to a boil, transfer to a baking dish and cover. Bake at 350°F for 45 minutes.

1. Heat oil in a large sauté pan over high heat.

2. Add onions and cook until tender.

3. Add rice and cook 8–10 minutes, stirring frequently, until toasted and brown.

4. Add garlic, cumin, mustard, cinnamon, bay leaf, salt, almonds, and apricots and cook another 5 minutes.

5. Stir in water and bring to a boil.

6. Reduce heat to low, cover, and cook 30–40 minutes, until liquid is absorbed and rice is tender. Fluff with a fork just before serving.

SERVES 4

430 calories
15 g fat
67 g carbohydrates
8 g protein
650 mg sodium
6 g fiber

INGREDIENTS
2 tablespoons olive oil
1 small yellow onion, chopped
1 cup brown rice
2 cloves garlic, minced
2 teaspoons ground cumin
1 teaspoon dry mustard
1 teaspoon cinnamon
1 bay leaf
½ teaspoon kosher salt
½ cup sliced almonds
1 cup dried apricots, chopped
1½ cups vegetable broth
1 cup water

Tabouli

This dish is a standard item on every Middle Eastern menu. Serve it with long spears of romaine lettuce and lots of lemon wedges.

1. Combine bulgur and water and soak for 30 minutes, until tender. Drain thoroughly.

2. In a large bowl whisk together lemon juice, salt, pepper, and olive oil.

3. Add parsley, onion, tomato, and bulgur. Toss to coat.

Which Wheat?
Cracked wheat has not been parboiled like bulgur and therefore must be cooked. To use it in this recipe, boil 2 cups water, reduce heat, add cracked wheat, cover, and simmer 15 minutes, until tender.

SERVES 4–6

160 calories
10 g fat
18 g carbohydrates
3 g protein
200 mg sodium
3 g fiber

INGREDIENTS
1 cup bulgur wheat
2 cups water
Juice of 1 lemon
½ teaspoon kosher salt
½ teaspoon ground black
    pepper
¼ cup olive oil
1 cup Italian parsley
1 small white onion, chopped
    and soaked in cold water
    for 15–30 minutes
1 large tomato, diced

Rosemary Roasted Yams

SERVES 8

280 calories
5 g fat
56 g carbohydrates
5 g protein
190 mg sodium
10 g fiber

INGREDIENTS
6 large yams, peeled and
    diced
2 large yellow onions, sliced
8 cloves garlic, peeled and
    left whole
3 tablespoons olive oil
¼ cup fresh rosemary
    needles, minced
½ teaspoon kosher salt
½ teaspoon black pepper

This is a fantastic dish on its own, but you can add some color to it with a diced beet or some purple potatoes.

1. Preheat oven to 400°F.

2. In a large bowl, combine yams, onions, and garlic.

3. Add the oil, rosemary, salt, and pepper and toss well to thoroughly coat.

4. Spread the vegetables out onto a cookie sheet in one single layer.

5. Bake, stirring occasionally, until tender and golden brown, about 1 hour.

Waldorf Salad

SERVES 4

340 calories
25 g fat
26 g carbohydrates
9 g protein
90 mg sodium
6 g fiber

INGREDIENTS
2 red apples, diced skin-on
4 stalks celery, diced
1 cup walnuts, toasted and
    chopped
1 cup green or red grapes,
    halved
1 cup light sour cream

This salad was created in the 1890s at the Waldorf Astoria Hotel in New York City. The original version used only apples, celery, and mayonnaise. Nuts and grapes appeared in recipes starting in the 1920s. We have lightened it up here with the help of light sour cream. Nonfat yogurt is another option, with slightly more tang.

1. In a large bowl combine the apples, celery, walnuts, and grapes.

2. Toss with sour cream to coat and serve chilled.

Which Apple?
You can use any apple you like in this recipe. It should be one that you enjoy eating out of hand. The Fuji is a personal favorite. This salad is also quite good when made with pears.

Chapter 11
Breaking Bad Habits

Poor nutrition is often a result of poor habits, developed throughout a lifetime, and encouraged by society. When you're caring for a family, it's especially important to have good eating habits, not only for yourself but also to provide a good example for your children. Poor eating habits can be kicked, but it won't happen overnight. This chapter includes all the information you need to know to kick bad habits (like skipping breakfast) and maintain healthy habits going forward.

The Most Important Meal

After twelve hours without nourishment, your body needs a fresh supply in the morning. Your blood glucose needs replenishment so that it can furnish the rest of your body with energy. Your brain, especially, needs glucose, as it has no capacity to store it. Eating breakfast helps your concentration, your ability to problem solve, your strength, and your endurance. What's more, intake of nutrients in the morning helps to regulate the appetite throughout the day, increasing your chances of meeting your daily nutritional requirements.

Breakfast is especially important for kids. A healthy breakfast improves overall cognitive skills, including memory, which gives them an edge in test taking, attendance, and class participation. Kids that skip breakfast tend to be disinterested, irritable, and lack the focus needed to succeed in class. And because a large chunk of their daily nutrients is missing, they tend to visit the school nurse more often.

Helping children develop a breakfast habit is likely one of the very best ways that parents can ensure lifelong success for their offspring.

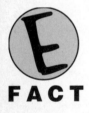

The Massachusetts School Nutrition Task Force reports a study in which students participating in school breakfast programs reported decreased trips to the school nurse, as well as increased math and reading scores, improved behavior, and attendance.

If that weren't enough to convince you to eat your breakfast, know that people who skip breakfast tend to be heavier. Hunger builds up as lunch approaches, and suddenly food is necessary, in any form. In this situation it is more common to throw caution to the wind and eat the first thing that presents itself. Overeating of the wrong foods is the result, and although the day is half over, the daily nutrient intake is far from half complete.

What's Your Excuse?

The general excuse for skipping the first meal of the day is lack of time. Busy lifestyles do not have to preclude health. You can eat a healthy breakfast in ten minutes or less if you plan for it. A bowl of cereal, a piece of fruit, and slice of toast is adequate.

Some people complain that breakfast upsets their stomach. Try to eat a small bit of fruit or bland toast each day, then slowly increase your intake as your system grows accustomed to it. It is possible that you have simply been choosing the wrong morning food for your sensitive stomach. You may also want to pack yourself a small breakfast snack and carry it with you for later in the morning, when your stomach is less sensitive, such as a nutrition bar or a piece of fruit.

What Is a Healthy Breakfast?

In general you want to eat foods of high nutritional value in the morning. Avoid sugary cereals, which have little nutrients. They raise your blood sugar quickly but then drop it way down to a point at which you are feeling hungry again within an hour. Fast food, too, should be avoided, as it is similarly short on nutrients, and generally contains excessive fat. Low-fat, low-sugar, high-fiber foods are the way to go. These foods help maintain your blood sugar level for hours and start your day with healthy nutrient intake.

Skipping Meals

Food is fuel. You need it for energy. When you don't eat, you lose energy. It's that simple. But today busy people find they do not always have time for meals. Unfortunately, it is almost impossible to get your daily recommended nutrients if you don't eat.

The daily nutrients are vital to the healthy functioning of all parts of your body. And although you may not notice when your body is running well, you certainly will notice when it starts to break down.

Good daily nutrition is the easiest way to achieve health and optimal performance. If you're not an Olympic athlete, you may wonder what optimal performance means for you. Brain function, cognitive reasoning, attentiveness, memory, and moods are all affected by nutrition. And the things you can't see, including a healthy immune system, are directly related to what you eat as well. Your body needs a constant flow of energy to run smoothly, and eating regularly is crucial to that end.

Fitting It In

As with all successful endeavors, planning is the key. If you typically don't have time for lunch, brown bag it and nibble when time allows. Energy bars, fruit, even a simple peanut butter and jelly sandwich provides an adequate supply of nutrients to get you through the afternoon.

When you skip meals, you are more likely to overeat the wrong foods at the next opportunity. Skipping midday meals leads to unhealthy binge eating in the afternoon and at dinner. Skipping dinner often leads to a similar fate late at night, and sleeping on a full stomach has its own negative impacts.

If time is your problem, planning is the key. Make an effort to shop weekly and stock your pantry with ready-to-eat or easy-to-prepare foods, such as whole-grain cereals and bread products, peanut butter, crackers, cheese, dried fruits, and nuts.

If you enjoy cooking, but are short on time, use your day off to prepare foods ahead of time. Chop herbs, onions, and vegetables and keep them in your freezer. Prepare sauces, and preportion meats. When you do cook, cook extra. Preportion meals and keep them in the freezer. When you're busy, you're more likely to eat if you have something ready to go than if you have to start from scratch.

To maintain a healthy eating schedule, routine is the key. Standardized menus may sound boring, but they make a lot of sense, especially if healthy eating is your goal. Shopping is easier and cheaper, and preparation becomes effortless. (Read more about menu planning in Chapter 16.)

Slowing Down

Overeating makes you overweight, and eating too fast is a big reason people overeat. When you eat, the food travels into your stomach fairly quickly. But it takes a full twenty minutes for your stomach to notice it's full, and to send that signal to your brain. In that time you are still feeling hungry, and the tendency is to overeat.

Eating slower improves your health and happiness in several ways. It makes you less likely to dive in for seconds, and less food in your stomach makes digestion easier. Plus, when you eat slower you can actually taste the food.

If you are prone to speed eating, there are a few tips you can try to slow down.

- Don't skip meals. Skipping meals is a common precursor to eating too fast.
- When you eat, sit at a table with a plate, napkin, and utensils. Don't eat while watching TV, and don't cram food into your mouth over the sink.
- Eat one forkful at a time, and put the fork down until the food is swallowed.
- Take sips of your beverage between each bite, and wipe with a napkin. Not only will you eat slower, but your improved manners will impress your friends and family.
- Make meals, especially dinner, a social event to share. Enjoy a conversation.

Eating is refueling, but it is also an important communal activity. It is especially important to show this aspect of mealtime to children. Teaching them to slow down, use manners, and enjoy the company at the table is an important lesson that will benefit them as they get older.

Controlling Portion Size

Hefty portions are another big contributor to overeating. Nutritional guidelines give you ample information regarding portions, but it can be a little intimidating. Visions of scales and measuring cups scare people away, and they go back to eating as much as they want. Unfortunately, when you combine large portions with speed eating, binging, and poor nutrition overall, the results are devastating.

This is not to suggest that measuring your food is not useful. But controlling your portion size does not need to include lab coats and beakers. A simple frame of reference is all you need. In general, most portions should resemble the palm of your hand. (Just the palm, not the fingers.) This is a good reference because everyone's palm is different, so variations in age and sex are simple to adjust for.

Don't serve food family style. Large dishes of food set on the table encourage overeating. Worse than that, family style can set up competition for the last piece, which results in speed eating (and sibling disputes).

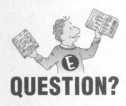

QUESTION?

What is family style?
Family-style service refers to large serving dishes set on the tables. Dishes are passed from person to person, each serving him- or herself. It provides the opportunity for second and third helpings, which means overeating. Instead, put the food on the plates in the kitchen, each with the intended portion.

One last trick to eating less is to serve food on smaller plate. Your eyes are definitely part of your eating experience. Seeing a tiny piece of food on a huge plate starts the meal off with disappointment.

Eating When You're Hungry

Physical cravings are a sign that your body needs food. But cravings can occur for other reasons, and it is important to understand the difference.

When your body is hungry, it tells you. Your stomach feels empty because it is. It growls and rumbles to tell you so. If you ignore it, you'll begin to feel lightheaded and tired and experience a loss in concentration or maybe even a headache. These signals are telling you to eat.

The delicious aroma of baking cookies is not a signal that it is time to eat. The beginning of a movie is not a signal that it is time to eat. Traumatic events are not a signal that it is time to eat.

If you are still unsure of the difference between wanting to eat and needing to eat, there are a couple of questions you can ask yourself. Can you wait it out? If you feel like eating but can wait until the next meal, you're not really hungry. If the feeling of hunger gets stronger as you wait, it's physical, not emotional, hunger.

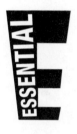

If you are craving a specific food, it is often a signal that your body is lacking in certain nutrients. You can tell if these are nutritional needs by examining your recent eating and activity pattern. Excessive salt, diminished protein, and extreme exertion can all result in food cravings as your body attempts to compensate.

Snacks

Snacking is not necessarily a bad thing, as long as it is sensible and adds to your daily nutritional goal. In fact, eating a few smaller meals helps digestion and is healthier overall than eating three larger ones.

Aim for a little bit of food every three to four hours. Snacks should be smaller than regular meals, and they should pack a nutritional punch. Make them low in fat and sugar. Plan them ahead of time, like you plan your meals, with nutrition in mind. Pack them to take with you so you are not tempted to hit the drive-through.

Avoid late-night eating. Although it may help you fall asleep initially, sleeping on a full stomach is not necessarily restful. The body doesn't digest well when sleeping, and conditions such as heartburn are more likely to wake you up. If you find that you are commonly awakened by hunger, a small healthy snack an hour before bedtime is a good idea. Unfortunately, most late-night eating is not healthy. It is binge eating of sweets or alcohol-related cravings that do nothing for you nutritionally. Schedules that include late-night work should include regularly scheduled healthy meals, with larger intake earlier in the day.

Caffeine and Alcohol

Except for water, coffee is the world's most consumed beverage. And wine grapes are the world's most abundant crop. But neither of these beverages, though they have significant cultural, social, and historical heritage, have much nutritional value. Caffeine is a stimulant, and alcohol is a depressant. Both of them alter the way your body functions, and both, when taken in excess, are damaging.

Caffeine

Caffeine is a naturally occurring substance found in the coffee bean, cocoa bean, kola nut, and tea leaf. Taken as a mild stimulant, caffeine increases body temperature, heart rate, and blood pressure. It restricts blood vessels to the brain, which prevents sleep, and causes the release of adrenaline, which makes you alert.

When abused, caffeine causes anxiety, stomach irritation, headaches, and insomnia. What's worse, it is addictive. Those who consume more than 300 milligrams a day will suffer withdrawal symptoms when cut off from their supply. Symptoms include fatigue, depression, irritability, jitters, and headaches as blood vessels in the brain dilate. Additionally, caffeine is a diuretic, flushing your body of fluids. This makes caffeinated beverages a poor choice as fluid replacements.

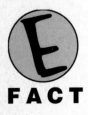

FACT

In addition to your favorite beverages, caffeine can also be found in some medications. Medicine for migraines often includes caffeine, which makes the drug work quickly. And caffeine is sometimes used to counteract drowsiness caused my certain medications, such as antihistamines.

Caffeine is not stored in the body, so its effects are not permanent. It can be felt ten to fifteen minutes after ingestion, and the effect lasts two to three hours. Tolerance for caffeine varies, but most adults should limit intake to

200–300 milligrams per day. One cup of coffee is about 90 mg, and sodas average around 40 milligrams.

Cutting Back

To cut back on caffeine, it's best to go slowly. Limit your caffeinated soda and tea intake, and switch your coffee to half-caffeinated. Then take heart in knowing that your headaches will disappear in a week or two.

Alcohol

Alcohol was first coveted as a way to purify water. But its virtues were soon eclipsed by its mind-altering effect and addictive properties. Alcohol is not in and of itself nutritious, and though certain forms may contain healthful properties, they are negligible in comparison to the damage they do.

Regularly consuming more than the recommended two drinks per day maximum (one for women) raises your chance of getting high blood pressure, stroke, and certain cancers, including liver, colon, esophageal, mouth, and breast cancer in women. Alcohol promotes dehydration, and it impairs muscle coordination, reflexes, reaction time, and balance. In addition, heavy consumption commonly results in malnutrition. While it does not contain many nutrients, alcohol does carry about seven calories for every gram. The calories replace those that would otherwise be consumed by nutritious foods, and alcohol inhibits the functions of many nutrients that are consumed.

Like all extras in your diet, alcohol should be used in moderation.

Eating Out

There are more restaurants than ever before. America has a booming food service industry, and food television programming has made people more aware of the culinary arts than ever before. With the variety of cultures that flourish in this country, you have a plethora of dining choices. But good nutrition requires you to examine the way you dine out.

Convenience Versus Social Dining

The next time you find yourself in a restaurant standing at a host's station, ask yourself why you are there. Is it because you are celebrating a special occasion? Are you spending some quality time with loved ones? Or are you simply looking for convenience over nutritional value?

Few restaurants are known for their nutritious meals. Yes, an occasional vegetarian or whole food establishment pops up from time to time, but these places are few and far between. Restaurants generally aim to attract a specific audience. Determining a restaurant's target audience is the first step in figuring out the healthiest places to dine.

Fine dining establishments are marketing toward the special occasion, or well-to-do diner. This is social dining. The experience is meant as a form of entertainment. A dining experience. Longer, more leisurely meals with multiple courses are a showcase for cuisine, and not necessarily meant to be well-rounded nutritious offerings. Prices usually reflect these targets, though quality doesn't necessarily follow. While these restaurants may not have particularly nutritious offerings on the menu, chefs in these establishments are more generally willing to fill special orders regarding less fat and salt. Here, too, you are more likely to find the kitchen using high-quality foods, including fresh, seasonal produce.

Theme restaurants can also be targeting the social diner, but here, the atmosphere is the main focus, not the food. This type of restaurant is less likely to have a healthy focus, and if the theme is geared toward kids, you will likely find even fewer healthy options.

Fast food, whether it be a worldwide chain, or a local taco stand, has only convenience to offer you. These restaurants focus on filling common cravings for fatty, salty, and sweet foods. They are located at convenient spots, including freeway off ramps, major intersections, grocery stores, and school campuses. Their goal is to get you to buy from them rather than cook for yourself, and so far, they have succeeded. People cook less than ever before. In fact, many kids grow up today never learning to cook. This trend is a dangerous one.

If you go to restaurants regularly, consider cutting back. Ideally, restaurants should be reserved for special occasions, but once a week is a good place to start. The health benefits of eating at home are substantial, and you'll save money, too.

Choosing the Right Restaurant

Healthy restaurant choices are not as important as healthy menu choices. Some of the world's healthiest cuisines, from places like the Mediterranean, Middle East, and Asia, also offer unhealthy choices. (Take the egg roll, for example. Delicious, but deep fried and full of oil.) But there are restaurants in which you are more likely to find healthy offerings. For example, restaurants with vegetarian menus are usually a good bet.

Asian cuisine typically emphasizes grain and vegetables and uses cooking methods that retain more nutrients. Mediterranean and Middle Eastern cuisines use far more grains and legumes and more monounsaturated olive oil. California cuisine is a trend from the 1970s that emphasizes fresh seasonal ingredients in a fusion of Latin American and Asian styles. It has a lot to offer in the way of nutrition, as does the latest trend of raw cuisine, in which food is barely cooked, if at all. But these cuisines can be just as bad as a bacon cheeseburger and fries if you don't choose wisely off the menu.

Healthy Menu Choices

Some restaurants, especially nationwide chains, have now begun to advertise healthful options. Low-sodium, low-fat, low-cholesterol, high-fiber, or "heart-healthy" options are clearly labeled, often with seals of approval from the American Heart Association.

Most places, however, do not have specialized menus, and it is up to you to know what to avoid. Steer clear of anything labeled "jumbo," "extra large," or similar phrases indicating enormous quantity. Chances are the portion is oversized. Don't order anything fried. Look instead for foods that are grilled or broiled. Ask for sauces and dressings on the side, and request that foods be cooked without butter or oil if possible.

Don't be afraid to ask for special orders. Most restaurants are used to it, and many chefs will happily replace your French fries with vegetables, salads, or fruit. Remember, restaurants need your business. They know that if they can please you, you'll likely return.

Chapter 12

Home Cooking

There's no place like home—for nutrition, that is. There is nothing better than a home-cooked meal made from fresh ingredients for your family's health happiness. If you already enjoy cooking, a change in ingredients is no big deal. But if you rarely set foot in the kitchen, you might need a little convincing. This chapter will help you get started preparing nutritious meals at home for your family.

Benefits of Cooking at Home

Cooking food at home is the single most important thing you can do for your health and the health of your family. When you do the cooking, you have control. You know exactly what everyone is eating. You control the quality and quantity, and you can cook to meet everyone's needs and preferences.

Cooking at home (meaning from scratch using fresh ingredients—not microwaving a frozen dinner) is fresher, which is a great start to more nutrients. You can maximize nutritional value by the cooking methods you use and by picking quality fresh foods without preservatives. You can also be sure of the cleanliness of the facility.

Eating out is fun, but it gets expensive. Home cooking from raw ingredients is not only healthier, it's also much cheaper. And you may find that cooking is just as fun as dining out, as well as rewarding and even therapeutic. No one says you need to make a feast fit for a king. There are simple dishes and simple preparations that are easy and satisfying.

Finally, there is no better way to show you care than to cook a healthy meal for your loved ones. It is a nurturing act that creates an enduring legacy. If you cook for your kids, they are more likely to cook for theirs, and so on. Good nutrition is a fantastic family tradition.

Healthy Cooking Methods

Preparation can dramatically affect the nutrient content of food. Cooking in a healthful way doesn't take much effort, but it does take some attention.

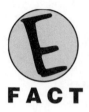

Sautéing, which comes from the French term meaning "to jump," is a similar technique to stir-frying. Foods are cooked quickly over high heat and kept in constant motion.

Broiling and grilling are known as dry-heat methods. They require no moisture, and little or no oil is necessary. Definitions vary, but grilling generally refers to food placed over a heat source, and broiling places food under a heat source.

The key to the success of dry-heat cooking is high heat. High temperatures seal the outside of the meat and hold in the juices. Lower temperatures allow more of the natural juices to drip out, yielding a drier finished product.

Stir-frying and pan frying require a small amount of oil. When using it for vegetables, the high heat limits the nutrient loss and keeps the colors fresh and bright.

Steaming is a moist-heat method. Food is suspended in a basket or perforated pan over simmering water, and the heat of the steam does the cooking. Unlike boiling, nutrients are not lost in the water. They can, however, dissipate into the air if overcooked.

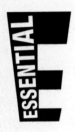

Poaching is great for delicate sausages, fish filets, quenelles, and delicate fruits. The liquid used can be flavored with herbs, spices, or aromatic vegetables, but it is meant strictly for cooking, and is not generally consumed.

Food can also be steamed in its own juices by wrapping it in foil or parchment paper and baking it in the oven. This is a particularly great way to maintain moisture and flavor for low-fat meats like chicken and fish.

Roasting is an all-around dry-heat technique that may or may not involve added fat. When used for meat, it is an excellent way to eliminate fat. Suspended on a rack above a roasting pan, the meat juices drip away.

Roasting is a great method for certain vegetables, including potatoes in their jackets, onions and garlic in their skins, and squash and pumpkin still in the rind. These foods essentially steam themselves soft, and their natural sugars concentrate, providing more natural flavor than when they are peeled and boiled.

Poaching is a moist heat method. It is not boiling, but it's close. Water is kept just below the simmer so that the food is not agitated by the motion of a rolling boil. Boiling employs water or other liquid brought to a rolling boil.

Food is added and cooked to the desired doneness. Simmering cooks the food under the boil, but still in motion.

Boiling not only increases the temperature of the cooking, but it keeps the food in motion. This is important for foods that tend to stick, like pasta. Because it leaches nutrients into the cooking liquid, it is best reserved for recipes that utilize the cooking liquid, such as soups and stews. Frugal chefs have been known to save cooking liquid for use in subsequent recipes. Stewing is another moist-heat method, and it usually refers to a longer cooking time. It also frequently refers to a liquid that thickens into a sauce as part of the meal.

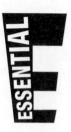

Stews are often enriched with fat or starch, and in most cases they include fatty meats. That's because this method works miraculously to soften the connective tissues of tough meats and melt away the fats, turning them into succulent tender delicacies.

Recipe Modification

Once you find the recipes you want to make, it may be necessary to adjust them to meet your current nutritional standards. This is not at all difficult, and it can be quite rewarding.

Altering recipes will rarely reduce the success of a recipe, although in some cases, it may take a few tries to get it where you want it. The best strategy is to change one element at a time, adding and subtracting methods that do and don't work.

Cutting Fat

Cutting fat is an easy alteration to make to any recipe. You can start by examining the raw ingredients.

Switching to leaner meat is easy. The fat content is generally displayed prominently on the packaging. You can switch to leaner beef or opt for chicken, turkey, or fish instead. Many recipes that are written for one type of meat can easily be made with another. Try turkey, salmon, or tuna burgers for a change of pace.

Oil can be used in place of butter in almost every circumstance. Olive oil is the healthiest choice, but the flavor is fairly prominent and not necessarily desirable in all circumstances. When you want a more neutral flavor, try peanut or canola oil instead. Don't even consider margarine. Even those with no trans fat have an elevated melting point, which leaves an unpleasant aftertaste in your mouth. Even with its saturated fat, butter is preferable to margarine. Another way to reduce the amount of fat in a recipe is to use a nonstick pan. Nearly every style of pot or pan ever manufactured comes in a nonstick version. Take care not to use metal utensils or scrubbies, or the nonstick surface will scrape off.

Choose reduced-fat cheeses, skim milk, light sour cream, low-fat cottage cheese, and nonfat yogurt. If cholesterol is an issue for you, replace eggs with egg whites or egg substitutes.

Cutting Sugar and Salt

There are many sugar substitutes available today, and many measure and cook up just like refined sugar. However, few have undergone any long-term study, and some can even produce unpleasant side effects. If avoiding refined sugar is your goal, consider using honey or date sugar. (Read more about sugar in Chapter 9.)

Sodium is easy to replace with salt substitutes (see recipes in Chapter 5). Eliminating it completely will take some getting used to, but it can be done successfully given time. Avoid adding salt to recipes until they hit the table to reduce the total amount of salt consumed. Reduced sodium products are plentiful, and many of your everyday salty groceries can be replaced by low-sodium counterparts. Check the labels, and compare brands.

Increasing Nutrition

Adding food with high nutritional value is a great way to improve your recipes. Increasing the amount of vegetables also increases the vitamins, minerals, and fiber. Try grating in squash, carrots, cabbage, chopped spinach, and fresh herbs to your next soup, stew, or casserole. Be sure to add these close to the end of the cooking to maximize their vitamin and mineral content.

Add dried fruits, seeds, and nuts to baked goods and grain dishes for added protein, vitamins, minerals, and omega-3 fatty acids. Sesame, flax, and walnuts are particularly healthful. Add legumes and whole grains to casseroles, soups, pasta dishes, and salads for added soluble and insoluble fiber and protein.

Pound for Pound

Certain products can, and should, be switched outright for use on a daily basis. Use whole-wheat flour instead of nutrient-challenged white all-purpose flour. Look for stone-ground organic varieties to maximize the nutritional value. You will find that your baked goods taste and look different, but take heart. You and your family will grow accustomed to it in short order. You may actually come to prefer it.

Shopping Strategies

Believe it or not, grocery shopping can be fun—if you are prepared and allot enough time for it, that is. It can also be a successful way to bring the entire family on board the healthy food express. Make them a part of the process and they are more likely to enjoy the changes.

Menu Planning

It may sound like a lot of work, and a little hyper-organized, but by planning out a week's worth of meals you will actually save time and money and eliminate a good deal of stress.

The first step is to brainstorm with your family for meal ideas. Remember that if they don't like it, they probably won't eat it. This is most important when it comes to snacking. If everything in the kitchen looks unappetizing, your family will find their snacks somewhere else.

After you have found recipes you like, make a list of all the week's meals, including breakfast, lunch, dinner, snacks, and dessert. Use it to make your list of ingredients. Whittle that list into the things you actually need to buy, then you're off to the races. (If you're a coupon clipper, don't forget them!)

Bring at least one helper to the market if you can. Kids will need lessons in label reading and price comparison. It may take a few trips until it sinks in, but persevere. Your goal is to teach them how to recognize the good from the bad. Be patient, and know that you are giving them valuable life skills.

A Healthy Pantry

Stocking your cupboards with food is not hard. Stocking with healthy food is a bit more challenging. Previous chapters have discussed how to pick nutritional elements. Now you need to be sure you have the right stuff on hand so that cooking healthfully is not a chore.

Have plenty of staple ingredients in the house. This includes whole-wheat flours, natural sweeteners, low-sodium broths, whole-wheat pasta, and plenty of fresh and frozen vegetables. Keep nuts and dried fruits on hand for snacking as well as recipes. Keep lots of seasonal fresh fruits and vegetables in the fridge, and if you have a farmers market, try to shop there from time to time for the really fresh, and often unusual, stuff.

Spices and Herbs

Keep plenty of flavorings around to add interest to your meals. Spices and herbs are a great way to do this. Spices are the bark, seed, resin, root, stem, fruit, or bud of a plant, tree, or shrub. They count among their rank the familiar, such as cinnamon, mustard, ginger, licorice, juniper, and cloves. Most are available whole and ground. They begin to lose their flavor and aroma as soon as they are ground, and the longer they sit on the shelf, the weaker they get. The most economical and flavorful way to purchase spices is in whole form. Spices kept whole will last for years with little loss of flavor and can be ground as needed. A mortar and pestle is the classic way to grind whole spices. There are also special spice graters and grinders at every gourmet gadget shop. But perhaps the easiest way to grind spices today is with a coffee grinder. Keep a separate grinder for your spices.

Some spices, especially seeds, benefit from light toasting prior to grinding to help release their aromatic oils. You can do this in a dry sauté pan on top of the stove. Keep the spices moving as they heat up, and remove them from the heat, and the hot pan, as soon as you smell the spice. Let the toasted spices cool down for a few minutes before you grind them. Larger spices, like nutmeg and cinnamon, can be broken into smaller pieces before being ground. A meat mallet is a perfect tool for this. If you're into gadgets, you can buy special graters designed especially for large spices.

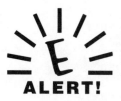

To get their maximum effect in your recipes, add spices early in the cooking process. Because fat is a natural flavor carrier, adding your spices to oil brings out the flavors and permeates a recipe.

Herbs

Herbs are green, leafy plants. With a few exceptions they have delicate, nonwoody stems. If allowed to grow to maturity, herbs develop into flowers and seeds. Many of these seeds are then reclassified as spices when dried.

You can use herbs in fresh or dried forms. They are usually interchangeable, but they each have different characteristics.

Dried herbs tend to have stronger flavor than their fresh counterparts, but they lose their flavor very quickly. Ground and powdered herbs have an increased surface area that allows the flavorful oils to dissipate faster. Buy them in small quantities and store them in a cool, dry, dark space to maximize their lifespan. When you're ready to use them, rub them in your hands to release more oils. Be sure to add dried herbs in the last thirty minutes of a recipe for maximum effect. In cold recipes, like salads and marinades, the longer the herb is in contact with the food, the more intense the flavor will be.

When choosing fresh herbs, look for bright green leaves that stay on the stem. You shouldn't see any bruised or dried leaves, and the stems should be straight. When you get them home, wash them right away, then drain them in a colander for a few minutes before refrigerating. Wrap them loosely in paper towels and store them in the produce drawer.

When adding fresh herbs to recipes, remember that you need more fresh herbs than dried. A general conversion rule is three parts fresh herb to one part dry. Chopping them very fine releases as much flavor as possible. Like any green vegetable, herbs discolor and loose nutrients when overcooked. Add them into recipes at the very end of cooking to maximize flavor and nutrients.

Homemade Flavorings to Stock in Your Pantry

You can buy all of these blends ready-made, but homemade is always more flavorful, and more rewarding. If you have a good assortment of whole spices and dried herbs, you can have these blends at a moment's notice.

Italian Blend

Use this seasoning blend in sauces, sausages, vegetables, or as a marinade rub.

Combine all ingredients in a large bowl and mix well. Working in batches, pulverize in a coffee grinder. Store airtight in a cool, dark place.

MAKES ABOUT 1 CUP

150 calories
6 g fat
18 g carbohydrates
6 g protein
30 mg sodium
10 g fiber

INGREDIENTS
¼ cup fresh chopped
   oregano
¼ cup fresh chopped basil
¼ cup ground fennel seed
2 tablespoons fresh chopped
   sage
2 tablespoons fresh chopped
   rosemary
3 cloves garlic, minced

Herbes de Provence

This classic blend can be made with fresh or dried versions of these herbs.

If using fresh herbs, mince all ingredients together and store airtight in the refrigerator. If using dried herbs, stir together and, working in batches, pulverize in a coffee grinder. Store airtight in a cool, dark place.

MAKES ABOUT 1¼ CUP

160 calories
3.5 g fat
33 g carbohydrates
10 g protein
35 mg sodium
15 g fiber

INGREDIENTS
¼ cup chervil
¼ cup marjoram
¼ cup tarragon
¼ cup basil
2 tablespoons thyme
2 tablespoons lavender

Fines Herbes

MAKES ABOUT ½ CUP

20 calories
0 g fat
3 g carbohydrates
1 g protein
10 mg sodium
1 g fiber

INGREDIENTS
2 tablespoons fresh parsley
2 tablespoons fresh chervil
2 tablespoons fresh chives
2 tablespoons fresh tarragon
2 tablespoons fresh
    marjoram

*Sprinkle these chopped fresh herbs onto seafood, poultry,
stews, soups, vegetables, or salads.*

Mince all ingredients together and store airtight in the refrigerator.

Chinese Five-Spice

MAKES ABOUT ⅔ CUP

140 calories
5 g fat
31 g carbohydrates
5 g protein
25 mg sodium
18 g fiber

INGREDIENTS
¼ cup black peppercorns
2 tablespoons fennel seeds
8 star anise
1 teaspoon whole cloves
2 cinnamon sticks

*This blend is commonly used to flavor
duck, chicken, pork, and fish.*

Combine all ingredients in a large bowl and mix well. Working in
batches, pulverize in a coffee grinder. Store airtight in a cool, dark
place.

Cajun Seasoning

This spicy blend adds New Orleans heat wherever you need it.

Combine all ingredients in a large bowl and mix well. Working in batches, pulverize in a coffee grinder. Store airtight in a cool, dark place.

MAKES ABOUT 3 CUPS

1,130 calories
37 g fat
197 g carbohydrates
47 g protein
125 mg sodium
87 g fiber

INGREDIENTS
1 cup bay leaves
1 cup paprika
¼ cup dried thyme
¼ cup dried oregano
¼ cup yellow mustard seed
¼ cup white peppercorn
¼ cup onion powder
¼ cup garlic powder
2 tablespoons cumin seed
2 tablespoons celery seed
*2 tablespoons cayenne
    pepper*

Garam Masala

Garam means "warm" or "hot," but this is not a spicy hot. Rather, it makes you feel warm after you've eaten it. Also, it's toasted prior to grinding. Use this whenever curry powder is called for, including in Chicken Madras, page 209.

Combine all ingredients in a large, dry skillet. Toast over high heat, stirring constantly, until fragrant, about 1 minute. Cool and, working in batches, pulverize to a fine powder in a coffee grinder.

MAKES ABOUT 2 CUPS

640 calories
30 g fat
102 g carbohydrates
20 g protein
160 mg sodium
42 g fiber

INGREDIENTS
1 cup bay leaves
½ cup cumin seed
¼ cup coriander seed
3 tablespoons black pepper
*3 tablespoons cardamom
    seeds*
3 tablespoons cloves
*3 tablespoons ground
    nutmeg*

Herb-Infused Oil

**MAKES ABOUT
1 QUART**

7,960 calories
877 g fat
39 g carbohydrates
13 g protein
95 mg sodium
25 g fiber

INGREDIENTS
1 cup fresh rosemary
1 cup fresh basil
1 cup fresh sage
4 cloves garlic
½ cup crushed fennel seeds
1 dried red chili pod
1 quart olive oil

*Infused oil is a quick and easy way to add flavor to a dish. Drizzle
it over pasta or use it to sauté vegetables or as a marinade. It can
also stand alone as a fantastic dip for crusty Italian bread.*

1. Finely chop rosemary, basil, and sage, and place in a sterilized glass jar.

2. Mince garlic and add to jar, along with fennel seeds and chili pod.

3. Cover with oil, being sure to submerge all ingredients. Seal with a sanitized lid and set aside in a cool, dark spot for two weeks. Shake jar daily to blend flavors.

4. When the flavor is infused, strain the oil into sterilized bottles and garnish with a clean sprig of rosemary.

Safety First
*Sterilizing jars keeps bacteria from forming. The easiest way to do this
is to run them through the dishwasher. You can also submerge them in
boiling water for 30 seconds. Be sure to sterilize both the jars and the
lids.*

Herb-Infused Vinegar

*You can use a single herb or spice to
create a terrific flavored vinegar.*

1. Finely chop parsley, chives, thyme, and tarragon, and place in a sterilized glass jar.

2. Add celery seed and set aside.

3. In a large sauce pan, bring vinegar to a boil.

4. At the boil, remove from heat and pour into jar with herbs.

5. Cover the jar loosely with cheesecloth or a towel and cool completely. Seal with a sanitized lid and set aside in a cool dark spot for two weeks. Shake jar daily to blend flavors.

6. When the flavor is infused, strain the vinegar into sterilized bottles, and garnish with a clean sprig of thyme.

**MAKES ABOUT
1 QUART**

**660 calories
15 g fat
110 g carbohydrates
20 g protein
160 mg sodium
17 g fiber**

INGREDIENTS
*2 cups fresh parsley
1½ cups fresh chives
1 cup fresh thyme
1 cup fresh tarragon
½ cup celery seed
1 quart white wine vinegar*

Chapter 13

Nutrition Plans for Moms

Good nutrition is always important. But if you're about to become a mom, or just considering it, this is the most important time to eat well. Not only does your developing baby need all the nutrients necessary for healthy growth, but you do too. In this chapter you'll learn all about prenatal nutrition.

Managing Weight Gain

Managing your weight gain during this time is critical for good health, both now and after the baby comes. A healthy weight gain during pregnancy should fall between twenty-five to thirty-five pounds. To keep your gain in check, continue to follow recommended dietary guidelines. (See Chapter 2 for more information about what to eat.)

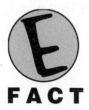

FACT

The phrase "eating for two" is corny, but it's true. Everything you eat is utilized for the growth and development of your baby. This includes the stuff you shouldn't have, as well as the stuff you should. In general, all doctors will tell you to eat a balanced diet, and to stay away from alcohol, tobacco, and caffeine, for your own health and that of your baby.

Concern for your nutrition should begin when the idea of a baby springs into your mind. Development begins at conception, and it may be several weeks before you get the good news. During those first weeks, cells are dividing, and the baby's brain and spinal tube (which will become the spinal cord) are already developing. To aid in this development, be sure to get enough folic acid, which should be obtained first through beans and dark, leafy green vegetables. It is also commonly fortified in foods such as cereals, and can be taken in a supplement. Aim for 230 mcg a day. Not all supplements contain folate, so check the label.

First Trimester

During this first period of pregnancy your weight gain should only be about two to five pounds. (If you begin pregnancy underweight, this number increases, and if you begin overweight, the number decreases.) Extra calories are not yet needed, but extra nutrients are. Make sure your food choices are nutrient dense (foods that are rich in nutrients and low in calories are considered nutrient dense). Keep your diet low in fat and full of whole grains and fresh vegetables and fruits.

In the first three months of pregnancy, a woman's hormone levels increase to ten times what they were prepregnancy. As you might imagine, it is especially important to consume nutrients connected with hormone production, such as vitamin C, vitamin B_5, calcium, chromium, and zinc.

Another challenge faced during the first trimester is keeping a balanced diet while experiencing morning sickness. This affliction doesn't only happen in the morning, nor does it always include actually getting sick. But it usually includes nausea, which makes getting your daily nutrients difficult. There are a few simple strategies to help keep your diet on track.

- Always have a little something in your stomach. Start the day with a plain starchy food, like crackers or toast, to give your stomach acids something to do.
- Eat smaller meals (five to six per day) every two to three hours, rather than three big meals per day. This ensures you are getting a steady flow of nutrients even if your meal pattern is interrupted by nausea and napping.
- Go ahead and nibble at night if you tend to wake up feeling nauseated.
- Avoid high-fat foods and fried foods. They are harder to digest, which can make your symptoms worse.
- Take any vitamin and mineral supplements you may be taking with meals. They can promote nausea on an empty stomach.
- Drink plenty of water to keep digestion flowing. If your morning sickness includes vomiting, be sure to replenish fluids and electrolytes that are lost.
- Queasiness is often triggered by smells, so avoid strong, disagreeable odors.
- Get enough rest, and nap when you need to.

Second Trimester

The fourth, fifth, and sixth months of pregnancy are commonly referred to as "the golden months." Morning sickness usually stops, and the discomfort of carrying a human being in your belly has not yet begun. You feel better and can finally eat the foods you have been too nauseous to enjoy.

Plan on gaining between nine and nineteen pounds in this period, or one to one and a half pounds a week. To achieve this feat, you will need to consume an extra 300 calories a day. Try to avoid getting these calories from a candy bar or a root beer float. Try adding a bowl of cereal and some fruit as a morning or afternoon mini-meal instead. Remember, you still need to maximize nutrients, because as your baby grows it consumes your nutrients.

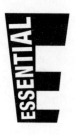

Make those extra calories high-nutrient foods. Extra vitamin C will help collagen production for developing tissues. Extra iron nourishes the placenta and increases your blood supply. (Remember, you need vitamin C to absorb iron.) Extra protein will help your baby grow one and a half to two and a half pounds during this time.

Keep exercising, especially if you were lying low the previous three months due to fatigue and nausea. And keep drinking water.

Third Trimester

During the last three months of pregnancy your baby will double in size. You may feel like you are too, but your weight gain should only be ten to eighteen pounds, or one to one and a half pounds per week. Don't be tempted to restrict your calorie intake. You and your baby need those calories for healthy development and strength. If you are feeling overweight, remember to make the calories count. Be mindful of adequate calcium and protein intake for growing bone and muscle tissue. If you are increasing protein, you may need more vitamin B$_6$ to aid in its digestion. Increased protein and less strenuous activity may induce periods of constipation. Be sure to eat plenty of fiber-rich foods, and even though you may feel as though you spend the entire day running to the bathroom as it is, drink lots of water to keep your system moving.

Continue to monitor iron intake (by being aware of the food you eat and making sure to eat foods rich in iron), and be sure you are getting enough omega-3 fatty acids and zinc, both of which help the baby's brain expand and develop. These nutrients, too, will help your body heal after the birth.

Cravings

Cravings are a normal, if exaggerated, part of pregnancy. With so many hormonal changes, and a heightened sense of smell and taste, it is no wonder moms-to-be crave foods. Over 75 percent of pregnant women report weird food cravings. They are most often for sweet foods, especially fruits, but can also include sour, salty, and spicy flavors. Go ahead and give in to these cravings because they are often an indication that your body needs something. Just be sure to combat these cravings in a healthy way. If you are craving a root beer float, it may be the sugar or the liquid your body wants. Try a juicy melon or peach, and see if that quenches your desires.

Along with cravings come the occasional food aversion. Foods you would normally consider delicious could make you feel queasy. When these foods include cheeseburgers or tacos there is nothing to worry about. If, however, the aversion is to spinach, it is important to substitute similar nutrients elsewhere in your diet. Odor can also trigger odd aversions, such as the smell of coffee. Don't worry, as your senses will eventually get back to normal.

Exercising for Two

Just as it was in your prepregnant life, exercise is an important part of over-all health now. If you have a regular exercise routine in place, keep it up, but check with your doctor to ensure it is not going to cause your baby any undue stress.

If you haven't been exercising regularly until now, it's a great time to start. You shouldn't take up rugby now, but gentle exercise is probably fine. Always check with your doctor to be sure.

Some great exercise options for pregnancy include walking, low-impact aerobics, swimming, cycling, or yoga. Be sure you do not do anything that could result in falling or injury. Stay out of excessive heat, and be sure to keep hydrated. (See Chapter 20 for more about exercise.)

Breastfeeding

Experts agree that, ideally, breast milk should be the baby's sole source of nutrition for the first six months, because it meets all nutritional needs for that period of growth. To provide adequate nutrients for both you and your baby, you should be taking in an extra 500 high-value calories each day. So, if you would typically be consuming 2,000 calories a day, you should be eating 2,500 while breastfeeding. If you have twins, the number can be increased to 3,000 calories. If you are already overweight, this number can be decreased.

Your diet should include more liquids, and extra calcium. The normal calcium recommendation is 1,000 mg per day, but lactating women should be taking 1,250mg. As during pregnancy, vitamins and minerals are all important. Remember that your baby is still developing.

Experimentation with solid foods can begin around four months, but only in very small quantities. Be sure not to offset regular breast milk feedings.

Solid Foods

It's not a good idea to start a baby on solid foods too early. The intestinal tract is not fully developed and solid foods are usually too much for young babies to handle. They are not able to swallow properly, and very young babies can't easily indicate they are full, which easily leads to overfeeding. Most importantly, starting solid foods too early can lead to the development of food allergies.

At four to five months breast milk should still be the sole source of nutrition. But it is fine to let the child get accustomed to a spoon, and a small amount of cereal mixed with breast milk can be used. Do not give more than one tablespoon a day before the age of six months. Baby rice cereal is a common choice, but ordinary oatmeal is far more nutritious.

By the age of six months, most babies are ready for new foods. Moving from breast milk to solid food is a delicate transition. If not done properly, weaning can lead to malnutrition.

When giving babies new foods, it is important to try only one food at a time for several days in a row before trying another. This makes it easier to detect allergic reactions, and it gives the child time to become accustomed to the food. Don't give up if the child's immediate reaction is negative. It can take several tries before a baby decides what it likes. Don't season the food, and don't mix foods until you are sure there is no allergy.

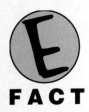

The flavor of breast milk is determined by the foods you eat. According to *The Journal of the American Dietetic Association*, if you have a healthy, varied diet, your baby will be accustomed to changes in flavor, and is less likely to be a picky eater.

Baby foods often contain too much water and not enough nutrients, especially protein and vitamins. Weaning diets are commonly deficient in vitamin A, iron, and zinc, the same nutrients that are of a concern during pregnancy. At six to seven months, as foods are introduced, it is important to continue breast milk to ensure babies are getting adequate nutrients.

Food Order

Controversy arises with the progression of foods. Many people feel that fruit is a bad starter food. Because it is sweet, it is thought that the child will grow to prefer sweet foods. This reasoning makes sense, although breast milk is also sweet. Bananas, avocados, yams, or sweet potatoes are commonly considered good first foods because their taste is similar to breast milk.

Meat is an important first food, because it is naturally high in protein and iron. Some feel that meat will trigger allergic reactions. But this is only a concern if the family has a history of such allergies. As long as foods are introduced one at a time, there is no cause for alarm.

Cereals can be increased, and new ones can be introduced. Millet is a good, high-protein option, as are whole-grain breads, and cereals. Cooked, strained, and mashed vegetables can be given at this time too.

Food Warnings

Several foods are off the list until after the first year, either because babies are not developed enough to handle them, or they are common allergens. Honey contains botulism spores that pass through older digestive systems but can create toxin-releasing bacteria in babies. Citrus is too acidic for baby's undeveloped digestive system. Cow's milk, eggs, wheat, corn, seafood, and soy are all potential allergens. Even after the first year, try new foods one at a time for several days in case of allergic reactions.

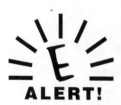
ALERT!

As with adults, there are some foods that should be avoided because they provide only empty calories and no real nourishment. Candy, soda pop, and caffeinated beverages act as stimulants, cause dehydration, and increase cravings in babies just as much as in adults. Introducing the things that you as an adult should be avoiding just doesn't make sense.

Growth Charts

Everyone looks different. But even though children all grow and develop at their own pace, parents want to know how their child is developing in relation to other kids. A growth chart can be an important tool in determining health.

Early nutrition plays an important role in the growth of children. Doctors monitor such growth by using a standard growth chart, developed by the Centers for Disease Control and Prevention (CDC). Using data gathered over a period of years from thousands of kids, a child's growth can be measured in percentile curves. The percentiles show the child's development in relation to other kids. For instance, if growth is in the twenty-fifth percentile, that means the child's growth is the same or more than 25 percent of kids in a similar population, and is less than 75 percent of kids in that same population. Higher or lower percentiles are not necessarily problematic. As long as the percentile follows the same pattern over time, growth is normal. It is only when the percentile changes dramatically that there can be cause for concern.

Pediatricians use growth charts to determine growth at the child's regular check up. Height, weight, and head circumference are measured and charted over time. There are a wide range of acceptable, healthy sizes for kids. Weight and height are determined by several factors, including genetics, lifestyle, nutrition, environment, activity, hormones, and overall health and well-being. Healthy, normal growth should continue along the same curve on the chart throughout childhood. Changes in the pattern, or movement off the curve, may signal health problems.

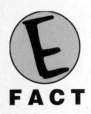

FACT

Girls and boys are measured on different charts because they grow and develop differently. There are also separate charts for children from birth to age three, from ages two through twenty, and special charts for kids with special needs.

For younger kids (under age three), height and weight should be increasing in proportion to each other. Head circumference maps brain development and generally does not change proportionally with height and weight. Older kids have their height, weight, and body mass index (BMI) measured. (See Chapter 20 for more information about BMI.)

Food Allergies

Food allergies occur when something enters the body, is perceived as a danger, and triggers an immune system response. Histamines are part of that response, which often manifests in respiratory and skin irritations.

You may have noticed a rise in allergies in recent years. Some schools are going as far as banning peanut butter because the problem is so severe. Foods must be labeled in clear, easy language if they contain foods that commonly have reactions. Luckily for allergy sufferers, many specialty products are tapping into the food allergy market. Even large chain restaurants are advertising items free of certain foods.

There are a few theories as to why so many people have food allergies today. Looking at human food consumption overall, some believe our global food supply is to blame, bringing foods from other parts of the world, from new sources with new allergens. Unrecognized allergens could also be occurring due to excessive manufacturing and high processing of foods.

Closer to home, it is thought that feeding baby anything other than breast milk in the first three months can damage the digestive system, suppressing the immune system and leading to food allergies. Our obsession with cleanliness is also a concern. Over use of antibacterial products may have weakened our immune systems by failing to challenge them.

The eight foods that are most likely to cause allergies are:

- Milk
- Eggs
- Peanuts
- Tree nuts (almonds, walnuts, cashews)
- Fish
- Shellfish
- Soy
- Wheat

If your child is at risk for food allergies or there is a history of food allergies in your family, it may be possible to prevent them. Combat this problem for your kids, before it becomes a problem, by following these steps:

- Feed only breast milk for the first six months. This means avoiding formula and any solid foods.
- While breastfeeding, mothers should avoid eating the top eight allergy foods, even if they are not themselves allergic.

- Follow the general solid food guidelines, offering only one food at a time, and for several days, before trying something new.
- Do not give milk, citrus, wheat, or eggs until age two.
- Do not give peanuts, tree nuts, fish, shellfish, or soy until age three.
- Keep a food log, and carefully record the foods your child eats and any reaction they produce. Even a mild reaction may be an indication of an allergy. Allergic reactions usually begin mildly and increase in severity with each subsequent exposure.
- As your child ages and foods become more and more processed, be sure to read labels carefully.

Chapter 14

Nutrition for Tots

When it comes to setting lifelong attitudes toward food, there is no more important time than the first few years of life. This time, between the breast and the school cafeteria, is your golden opportunity to shape the food habits of your child. This chapter covers nutritional information for kids ages two to five.

Starting Early

You can give a child solid foods as early as six months of age, but it is not until the second year that regular patterns of eating take hold. Year two is also a time ripe for problems to arise. As children begin sitting and eating with family, eating patterns begin to change, social cues are learned, and behaviors are enforced. The more you know before you start, the fewer problems you will have feeding your child down the road.

As children grow it is the parent's job to help them become independent eaters so that eventually they will take the responsibility for their own nutrition. The earlier the quest for independent eating begins, the more successful it will be. There are some very easy things you can do to get your children off on the right foot:

- Be an example. Eat a wide variety of healthy foods in sight of your child. Avoid the foods you want your child to avoid.
- Set a schedule. Well-spaced meals and snacks at regular times make for happy tummies and help avoid the empty, hungry feeling that is typically accompanied by whining and lack of cooperation.
- Teach your kids that food is fuel. Like gas in the minivan, it gives us energy to get through the day. Do not teach that food is a reward, a weapon, a punishment, or a substitute for love.

First Whole Foods

As discussed in the last chapter, there are several theories regarding what is the best progression of solid foods. The fact is that as long as you take the foods one at a time, and are mindful of balancing the diet, the order of foods isn't important. However, as your child begins to feed himself, new considerations must be taken into account, especially the dangers of choking.

Hot dogs and grapes are the all-time leading choking foods, along with nuts, raw carrots, popcorn, and hard candies. The size and shape are just right for lodging in the trachea and blocking airflow through it.

Most of these foods are not recommended for young children anyway, so by following a sensible diet, your child is already better off. While few children are allergic to hot dogs, they are not a good source of protein. Yes, they are easy to eat, mild, and most kids gobble them up. But they are loaded with saturated fat, sodium, and sugar. Children are better off eating boiled chicken or turkey.

Trying New Foods

Continue to introduce new foods to your child, but do not force them. This is a period when food plays an important role, both good and bad, in your child's life. It can make her feel more grown up, or give her control over you. Be very careful!

To introduce something new to a toddler, place no more than one or two tablespoons of it on the plate. Do not announce it or let them know it is new. Do not watch in anticipation, or warn them they may not like it. Just sit down and eat it too. If they don't like it, and many will not, let it go for this meal, but try it again another night. Sometimes it takes a dozen tries before a child will try something new. The key is to not make a fuss about it. If this refusal to eat gets attention, the behavior will continue, even if the attention is negative.

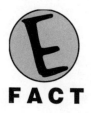

Distaste and fear of food contamination is common in toddlers. It could be a natural survival mechanism, meant to prevent recently mobile kids from eating everything in sight. Foods that look, smell, and taste weird are often immediately rejected.

New foods or textures mixed into familiar foods are frequently detected because a child's palate is more sensitive than an adult's. Not only will the food be rejected, but the parent will lose trust.

Foods that the child believes resemble something gross (such as noodles that look like worms) may be rejected. Often, anything touching the "worms," or merely on the same plate, will also be rejected by association. Forcing the issue in cases like this can make matters much worse, leading to retching and vomiting. Letting matters get to this point has the potential for a long-term negative association with that food, and the battle is lost.

Ban the Bland

There is no scientific evidence that suggests children cannot tolerate spicy food. This is a culturally determined phenomenon, and can be demonstrated by observing cultures known for their spicy cuisine. Children in these cultures do not eat different food than their parents. Why do American children?

If you dislike spicy foods, chances are your child will also grow up disliking or at least not going out of his way to consume them. This is true with everything you dislike, simply because chances are slim that you will cook food for the family that you will not eat yourself.

But if you enjoy interesting, flavorful foods, there is no reason not to share them with your child. It may not be immediately appreciated, but over time, with repeated exposure, it will become part of their ever-expanding culinary repertoire.

In this same vein, there is no reason children must eat "children's food." Starting off by preparing separate meals for separate members of the family sets a bad precedent, guaranteeing you more work down the road. If the adults are eating a balanced meal, the kids can share in it. Eating adult food with adults will expose children to a variety of tastes and nutrients, and it begins the important education in manners.

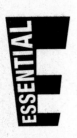

Food jags are a common occurrence with kids of this age. A jag is when they insist on eating only one food for breakfast, lunch, and dinner. They can last for a week or two, but there is no need to worry about malnutrition. If it goes on longer, help break the cycle by including them in the shopping and cooking.

Picky Eaters

A baby's weight triples in the first year, and then the rate of growth drastically slows in year two. It will take at least another year until he reaches four times his birth weight. Yet parents often continue to feed their children at the same rate. The kids know they don't need as much, because they just aren't hungry, and so begins the tug of war that is mealtime. Forcing children to eat, over-feeding, and putting too much emphasis on cleaned plates is a clear contributor to the 25 percent of two-year-olds nationwide that are at risk for obesity.

This is the time parents must draw a distinction between picky eating, and just plain not hungry. In most cases, when children of this age are hungry, they will eat. If they taste a food and reject it, don't force the issue. It is negative attention to eating that initiates the poor food relationships that can last a lifetime.

Kids that don't eat are a constant worry to their parents. The fear of malnutrition makes parents constantly offer their kids food. But the root of the loss of appetite is usually the parents' fault. Often kids are given too much milk and juice. Toddlers should not be drinking more than sixteen ounces of milk a day, and no more than four ounces of 100 percent juice. Parents should also limit snacking, especially sweet snacks. If they are filling up on these things throughout the day they will have very little appetite when family mealtime rolls around.

Portion size is another area of concern. Kids do not need adult portion sizes, but it is adult portion sizes that are on food labels. Chapter 2 told you to relate your portion size to the palm of your hand. The same is true for a toddler. Look at his hand and use it to judge portion size. If you want to be more precise, a toddler should be getting about 1,300 calories a day, or 40 calories per inch of height. This is about one-quarter of the food the parents eat.

To help ensure those 1,300 calories mean something nutritionally, use the following guideline, based on the dietary recommendations in Chapter 2:

Toddler Dietary Guidelines

Food	Toddler Servings
Whole Grains	6
Vegetables	3
Fruit	2
Milk	2
Meat/Protein	2

Don't Force It

Forcing kids to eat when they are not hungry not only sets up dislike for foods, but dislike for mealtime as well. If they do not appear to be eating a balanced diet, watch the intake throughout the week before you jump to conclusions. Many kids will make up for lost nutrients within a period of several days. If it is still a concern, discuss vitamin supplements with your pediatrician. In most cases, chances are good that your child will eat the amount of food he needs. As long as growth is continuing along the normal pattern there is no need for alarm. (Read about growth charts in Chapter 13.)

Kids also eat poorly for external reasons. Loss of appetite commonly occurs with fatigue and illness. Sore throat, fever, teething, constipation, or gastrointestinal distress can cause loss of appetite. If kids are anxious, sad, or lonely, they may not want to eat. If they are distracted by the television, they may not eat well.

Eating with the Family

Sitting down to a family meal is one of the most important habits you can initiate for your child. You'll reap the benefits now, and even more so during the teen years. Studies have shown that children who eat at the family table on a regular basis get better grades and are less likely to smoke, do drugs, drink alcohol, suffer depression, have eating disorders, or commit suicide, and they are more likely to delay having sex. If that's not enough for you to set the table, consider it a great way for them to learn manners, engage in conversation, and learn what it means to be civilized.

Before the Victorian era, mealtime was a blessed refueling. Unless you were part of the aristocracy, everything you did was in pursuit of food for your table. Agriculture, hunting, trading, and arts and crafts were all means of putting bread on the table. And when the bread made it to the table, people were thankful. Food was sacred and life-giving, and in many cases, eating it was ceremonial.

Recreational eating became commonplace after World War II, as did the dinner party. The family dinner was fully ingrained by the 1950s but began to disappear in the following decades, as single-parent families and two-income households became the norm. Fast food and microwaves taught us that we had better things to do than cook. Television and overbooked schedules gave the kids better places to be than the table. The ceremony of mealtime was gone.

Now that food is easy to acquire (you don't even need to leave your car), people no longer take the time to be grateful. They shovel it in and move on. But the ceremony of meals is still important. And the earlier this ritual begins, the more benefit your child will receive from it.

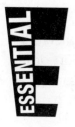

Social cues and citizenship are learned at the family table. Kids learn big words and how to talk conversationally. They learn to pass the salt and share and compromise. They learn which fork to use, how to eat what is put in front of them, and how to stay seated politely until everyone is done.

Dinnertime is a great opportunity to learn about your family's day. Togetherness is the focus. It should be a time anticipated by everyone, not dreaded or avoided. Only the parents can create this environment, but the kids can help. Give them chores at a very early age. Setting the table or, for the very young, just setting out napkins is a start. Older kids can create placemats or name cards, make centerpieces, and even create and cook the meal.

Working with Child Care Providers

If your child is in child care, chances are good that she receives at least one main meal and one snack from the child care provider. If you're concerned about early childhood eating conditions, make this an essential part of your initial search for a provider.

Be sure they are feeding your child foods you approve of and that the eating environment is relaxed, sanitary, and well planned. Use this checklist when shopping for childcare:

❑ Who plans the meals?
❑ Do they follow the Food Guide Pyramid?

- [ ] What foods are served?
- [ ] Take a look at the kitchen. Is it clean?
- [ ] Are foods stored properly?
- [ ] Who prepares the meals?
- [ ] Do the adults have safety and sanitation training?
- [ ] Do the menus include whole grains and fresh vegetables and fruits?
- [ ] Do they serve milk?
- [ ] Is the juice 100 percent juice, or does it contain high-fructose corn syrup?
- [ ] Do they serve fried foods, such as chips?
- [ ] Is mealtime pleasant?
- [ ] Does a caregiver sit with the children?
- [ ] Are the children relaxed during mealtime, or is there stress?
- [ ] Are records of intake kept for each child so parents can keep track?

Recipes for Tots

The following recipes are designed to be nutritious and tasty to both kids and adults, but with a particular youthful slant. The idea is for the entire family to eat the same meal.

Cheesy Eggs

*This recipe is warm and creamy, and it introduces the fla-
vors of herbs and cheese, as well as the textures of eggs and
melted cheese. Fines herbes is a terrific blend because it is
subtle but distinctive. There is no salt added to this because
young palates don't need it. You may want to set the table
with salt and pepper for the grownups.*

1. Heat olive oil in a nonstick sauté pan over high heat.

2. Whisk together egg, cheese, and herbs, and add to the hot pan. Stir
   immediately and quickly, until the egg is no longer wet, about 1
   minute.

3. Turn off heat and let sit for 30 seconds to completely melt cheese. Serve
   immediately.

Fines Herbes

*This French herb blend is terrific sprinkled onto seafood, poultry, stews,
soups, vegetables, or salads. You can buy it ready-made or make it
yourself by blending equal parts fresh chopped parsley, chervil, chive,
and tarragon.*

SERVES 4

121 calories
9 g fat
1 g carbohydrates
8 g protein
116 mg sodium
0 g fiber

INGREDIENTS
½ tablespoon olive oil
4 eggs
*¼ cup sharp Cheddar cheese,
    shredded*
*1 tablespoon Fines Herbes
    (Page 156)*

Yogurt and Fruits

Some kids love sour foods. Others take some time to warm up to them. Yogurt mixed with naturally sweet fruits is a great introduction to the tangy side of life.

Choose a variety of sweet seasonal fruits in an assortment of colors, like bananas, pears, strawberries, and melons. Cut them into bite-size, finger-grabbing pieces, toss with yogurt, and serve. Alternatively, you can serve the yogurt on the side, if your kids like to dip.

Added Sugar
You may consider adding a touch of honey to sweeten the mix. But stay away from presweetened yogurt. The added sugar does more harm than good.

SERVES 2

30 calories
0 g fat
7 g carbohydrates
1 g protein
15 mg sodium
0 g fiber

INGREDIENTS
¼ cup plain nonfat yogurt
¼ cup mixed seasonal fruits

Noodle Salad

These traditional Asian flavors are loved the world over. Associating them early with fresh vegetables and whole-grain noodles is preferable to the association they'll pick up later with deep fried mall food and heavily sweetened, starchy sauces.

1. Bring a large pasta pot of water to a boil over high heat. At the boil, add pasta, and stir until the boil resumes. Cook until tender, but al dente. Drain, rinse with cold water, and set aside.

2. In a large bowl, whisk together garlic, ginger, sesame oil, soy sauce, peanut oil, and rice vinegar. Add carrot, zucchini, pepper, sesame seeds, and cooked pasta. Toss well to thoroughly coat. Serve chilled or at room temperature.

Al dente
This is an Italian term that means "to the tooth," and refers to the degree to which certain foods, usually pasta and vegetables, are cooked. These foods are cooked until done, but still have slight texture when bitten. They are not raw or crunchy, nor are they soft.

SERVES 4

270 calories
7 g fat
47 g carbohydrates
10 g protein
270 mg sodium
9 g fiber

INGREDIENTS
½ pound whole-wheat
    spaghetti
1 clove garlic, minced very
    fine
1 teaspoon grated ginger
1 teaspoon sesame oil
1 tablespoon soy sauce
1 tablespoon peanut oil
2 tablespoons rice vinegar
1 carrot, grated
1 zucchini, grated
1 red bell pepper, diced fine
1 tablespoon sesame seeds

Tofu Stir-Fry

Tofu is an excellent source of protein, and an early appreciation for it will open up all sorts of culinary doors. Tofu picks up the flavors that surround it and this savory sauce is perfect. If you are avoiding peanuts, replace the peanut butter with almond butter.

1. In a small bowl whisk together water, peanut butter, vinegar, soy sauce, honey, and cayenne pepper. Set aside.

2. Heat wok or sauté pan over high heat and add oil. Add garlic and ginger and cook, stirring, until browned.

3. Add tofu and continue to cook 3–5 minutes, stirring, until browned.

4. Add scallions and broccoli and cook until tender and bright green.

5. Add prepared sauce and stir to warm through. Serve immediately over brown rice.

SERVES 4

370 calories
27 g fat
17 g carbohydrates
23 g protein
430 mg sodium
5 g fiber

INGREDIENTS
½ cup water
½ cup peanut or almond
    butter
¼ cup rice or cider vinegar
1 tablespoon soy sauce
1 tablespoon honey
¼ teaspoon cayenne pepper
1 tablespoon canola oil
2 cloves garlic
1 tablespoon grated ginger
1 pound firm tofu, diced
1 cup scallions, chopped
2 cups broccoli, chopped

Chapter 15

Nutrition for Elementary-Age Children and Preteens

School, sports, scouts, friends, and family are all vying for your children's attention. They have a hundred different things to occupy their time, a hundred things they want to try, and a hundred ways to get into trouble. They have developed their own distinctive personality, and they are probably not afraid to tell you what they think. Are they thinking about food? You bet. Are they thinking about nutrition? That depends on you.

How Much Is Enough?

Until they reach age three, kids will typically eat only as much as they need. But as they age, they begin to eat things for pleasure. This sudden change can, if left unchecked, lead to childhood obesity. Kids, like adults, should not eat more than they need to fuel themselves.

Portion Size

As at any age, the palm of the hand is still a good indication of portion size. Beginning at about age five, and until age nine or ten, kids need about half the amount of food that adults eat. (See Chapter 2 for more about portion size and dietary requirements.) Thus, it is important to refrain from serving them the same size portions as the grownups get. If you put that much food in front of them, they will probably eat it, and this will lead to unnecessary weight gain.

When and What Kids Should Eat

Breakfast, lunch, midmorning and afternoon snacks, and dinner should fulfill a child's nutritional needs if they follow the dietary guidelines laid out in Chapter 2. But skipping meals, excessive snacking, and lack of exercise can throw a kid's diet out of balance.

Breakfast is the most important meal for school-age kids as well as adults. If kids are hungry midmorning, they will have poor concentration and difficulty with brain function. Breakfast does not need to be limited to traditional breakfast foods. It's worth taking time to find nutritious foods they'll eat willingly, rather than to fight through the meal, or let them skip it.

A brown bag is preferable to a school cafeteria lunch. School lunches are typically packed with fat, sodium, and sugar and are overcooked to the point of diminished nutrient content. They usually don't taste very good, and they can do some damage to the positive food attitudes you have been trying to build. Select what goes into the brown bag with care. By lunchtime they will be hungry and will need healthy energy, not sugar-packed juice drinks and junk food.

By dinnertime, if they have been eating nutritiously in appropriate quantities all day, they will probably be ready to clean their plates. One way to ensure they'll eat what's put in front of them is to make sure they get a daily dose of vigorous exercise to round out the day's healthy activities.

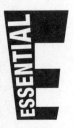

Snacks are a useful way to stave off hunger and to ensure all daily nutrients are being consumed. But this only works if the food is nutritious, so keep healthy snacks in the house. High-fiber, low-sugar snacks are ideal and provide enough stamina to get through the homework without nodding off from a sugar crash. Veggie sticks, cheesy popcorn, and cereal are excellent choices.

Food and School

When kids enter school they are confronted with new experiences and challenges, many of which include food and eating. Here, among their peers, pressure to fit in begins, often in the lunch room. Even if you pack their lunch, there will be the inevitable trading, bargaining, and auctioning off of sweet snack cakes and candy. It is important to arm your school children with nutritional smarts.

They should know what constitutes a healthy diet before they lay eyes on the lunch lady. Teach them which foods will make them fat, tired, or sick, and which foods will make them strong and healthy. Before they enter school, get them used to skim milk, vegetables, fruits, and whole grains. Limit the extras like ice cream and candy. Sweets should be fruit, and desserts should be reserved for special occasions.

The food you send to school should be as healthy as the food they eat at home. Avoid prepackaged lunches. They are typically loaded with sodium, fat, and sugar. The lunch line may not be much better. Remember that even if the school offers "healthy" choices, there is no guarantee it's what the kids will pick.

Tackling Persnickety Kids

After age five, parents no longer need to worry about the adequate calorie intake of their children; as noted, the problem lies in limiting caloric intake. That is why it is particularly important to monitor the quality of the calories and the way they conduct themselves at the table.

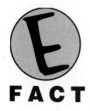

Sixty percent of American toddlers eat pastry every day. Ten percent of American babies four to six months old consume sweets, including soda pop. Baby food companies do not put sugar in their fruits and vegetables, but they do sell baby dessert. Remember, a child's sweet tooth is easily placated by fruit.

If you find yourself with a difficult eater, there is no need to bend over backward. Part of growing up is learning to eat politely, and show respect. As a parent, you should not tolerate persnickety behavior. But in keeping with the calm, stress-free idea of the family table, try not to let the pickiness instigate conflict. To combat your persnickety kid, here are a few tips:

- Be upbeat and calmly explain that they are expected to taste everything. If they do not like it, that's fine, but there will be no more food offered that evening.
- Don't force the plate clean. Don't badger them to eat it. Food taste is a very personal thing. What is perfectly acceptable to one may be not at all pleasant to another. Arguing over it is pointless. You can ignore it or simply state, "Too bad. Maybe someday you'll like it."
- Do not make multiple meals. You are not a short-order cook. If they are hungry, they will eat.

Encouraging Experimentation

One of the greatest things about food is the immense variety of it. Kids that are offered a wide variety of foods during weaning are less likely to be persnickety older children. By age five they are old enough to try new cuisines, both out on the town, and in the comfort of home.

One way to interest kids in new foods is to interest them in the place it came from. Go to a map and pick a country. Or pick something they're interested in and look for related foods.

If your kid likes ancient Egypt, find out what Egyptian cuisine is all about. If your kid likes music, learn about the food eaten in the music capitals of Nashville (BBQ), New Orleans (Cajun/Creole), or Mozart's Austria (schnitzle and Sacher torte). If it's sports they love, learn about the native culture of favorite players, or the famous food of the team's hometown. Every subject can somehow be related to food in a fun and interesting way.

Childhood Obesity

Our industrialized society of sedentary jobs and high-calorie, low-nutrient convenience food has created an epidemic of obesity. Since the mid-1980s, the number of overweight children ages six to ten has doubled. For teens, the number has tripled. The result is a generation of children battling diseases that were once thought to belong to adults: diabetes, high blood pressure, and high cholesterol.

To battle the epidemic, families must improve diet and exercise together. Set a good example. Children will naturally want to eat when they are hungry, but eating because they are bored is a learned behavior.

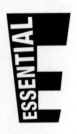

Be careful to avoid giving food a role in behavior modification. It should be neither given as a reward for good behavior nor withheld as punishment for bad behavior. Consider rewarding kids with outings, or activities, and make punishment relevant to the crime, not the dinner table.

It is also important to monitor the scrutiny you give your child's eating behavior. Not enough attention can lead to poor habits, but too much can lay the ground work for eating disorders. Discuss health and fitness, but try to build self-esteem by being positive, not critical. Focus on attainable fitness levels as goals, such as the number of laps to swim or miles to bike. Celebrate achievements, even little ones, but not with food.

Recipes for Lunchboxes and Snacktime

No healthy lunch program will ever deliver what your brown bag does. Plus, you pack it with love. Yes, it takes time. And yes, it takes planning. Most things worth doing do. Let your child help in the planning and the making. While it may take some training initially, it will make it easier on you in the long run, and your child will have much more invested in the lunch he chose and made.

Mini Hero Sandwich

MAKES 1 SANDWICH

540 calories
35 g fat
31 g carbohydrates
29 g protein
1,480 mg sodium
4 g fiber

INGREDIENTS
1 whole-wheat hot dog bun
2–3 slices chicken or turkey
2 ounces sliced cheese of
    your choice
½ cup shredded lettuce
1 thin slice red onion
2–3 slices tomato
2–3 slices cucumber
1 radish, chopped
1 tablespoon olive oil
1 tablespoon red wine
    vinegar
1 teaspoon Italian seasoning

This sandwich really is a hero because it has been trimmed of much of its fat and sodium. For healthiest results, use leftover roasted chicken or turkey instead of processed lunch meats. You can even make this with tuna or egg salad.

1. Slice bun in half lengthwise, leaving one edge intact, like a hinge.

2. Open up the roll, and arrange the meat and cheese evenly.

3. Place the lettuce and assorted vegetables evenly down the center of the open roll.

4. Drizzle with olive oil and vinegar and sprinkle with Italian seasoning.

5. Close the roll back up, slice in half, and wrap tightly in wax paper.

What's in a Name?
The hero is the New York name for this sandwich. In Philly it's a hoagie, throughout New England it's a grinder, in Connecticut it's a submarine, and in Maine it's an Italian. Stack it higher for a Dagwood.

Baby Bagel Sandwich

This is the cutest, tastiest peanut butter sandwich in town.

1. Slice open the bagel and spread peanut butter on each half.

2. Stick raisins in the peanut butter of one half, and bananas in the peanut butter of the other half.

3. Close it and wrap it tight.

Jelly-Belly
Sure, jelly is the normal accompaniment to peanut butter, but it's loaded with sugar. If your family is into jelly, choose a sugar-free, or fruit-only spread instead. No one needs that extra sugar.

MAKES 1 SANDWICH

310 calories
17 g fat
32 g carbohydrates
11 g protein
280 mg sodium
4 g fiber

INGREDIENTS
*1 mini bagel
2 tablespoons peanut butter
2–3 wheels of banana
1 tablespoon golden raisins*

Tiny Cracker Sandwiches

Who says sandwiches have to be on bread? These little nibbles are cute enough to serve in Barbie's dream house.

1. Place 4 crackers on a plate.

2. Layer with cheese, radish, cucumber, a dot of mustard, and top with a second cracker.

3. Pack them in a small plastic container to hold them together until lunchtime.

Sodium Watch
Look for lower sodium crackers and mustard to keep this little lunch from getting too salty. Excess sodium in a kids' diet can increase dehydration, and prime their palate for the saltier side of life.

MAKES 4 MINI-SANDWICHES

150 calories
11 g fat
6 g carbohydrates
7 g protein
230 mg sodium
< 1 g fiber

INGREDIENTS
*8 whole-wheat crackers
4 small squares of cheese
4 small wheels of radish
4 small wheels of cucumber
1 teaspoon mustard*

Pita-Hummus Pockets

MAKES ABOUT 2 CUPS
HUMMUS, ENOUGH
FOR A WEEK OF SAND-
WICHES

160 calories
6 g fat
26 g carbohydrates
5 g protein
250 mg sodium
4 g fiber

INGREDIENTS
1 (15-ounce) can chickpeas
    (reserve liquid)
2 cloves garlic
½ medium yellow onion,
    chopped
2 tablespoons tahini
2 tablespoons lemon juice
¼ cup olive oil
½ teaspoon ground black
    pepper
1 circle whole-wheat pita
    bread
5–6 slices cucumber

Hummus is a staple item in every Middle Eastern household and is generally used as a dip for flat bread. It is delicious, satisfying, and packed with protein.

1. Combine chickpeas, garlic, onion, tahini, lemon juice, and olive oil in a food processor and puree.

2. Add enough reserved chick pea liquid to reach a smooth, yogurt-like consistency.

3. Season with pepper.

4. Slice pita in half and open pocket. Fill each half with cucumber slices, and 2–3 tablespoons hummus.

5. Wrap each half tightly in wax paper.

Portion Control
One half of a pita sandwich is sufficient for a kid's lunch. If you're only making lunch for one, wrap the remaining pita and keep it in the freezer until the next day. Bread stays fresher when frozen.

Chicken-Caesar Wrap

1. In a large bowl, whisk together the egg yolk, garlic, anchovies, and lemon juice.

2. Slowly drizzle in the olive oil while whisking, taking 3–4 minutes to add all the oil.

3. Stir in Parmesan cheese, then set aside.

4. Lay the tortilla flat, fill with lettuce and chicken, and drizzle with dressing. Fold side edges of the tortilla toward the center, then roll up from the bottom. Wrap tightly with waxed paper.

Something's Fishy

Many people feel that anchovies make the Caesar dressing complete—without them, it just doesn't taste right. The full, salty flavor really rounds out a recipe, but should never stand out and be noticeable. As an added bonus, anchovies are powerhouses of nutrition, high in calcium, niacin, iron, and protein.

MAKES ABOUT 2 CUPS DRESSING, ENOUGH FOR A WEEK OF SAND-WICHES:

per wrap
202 calories
7 g fat
20 g carbohydrates
19 g protein
307 mg sodium
2 g fiber

INGREDIENTS
1 egg yolk
1 clove garlic, minced
4 anchovy filets, minced
3 tablespoons lemon juice
¼ cup olive oil
½ cup freshly grated Parmesan cheese
1 whole-wheat tortilla
½ cup romaine lettuce, chopped
⅓ cup boneless chicken, cooked

Pasta Salad

SERVES 6

300 calories
13 g fat
40 g carbohydrates
11 g protein
350 mg sodium
6 g fiber

INGREDIENTS

2 tablespoons red wine
vinegar
2 cloves garlic
1 tablespoon Italian
seasoning
¼ cup olive oil
1 scallion, chopped
1 ripe tomato, diced
1 red bell pepper, diced
1 pound whole-wheat pasta,
cooked and cooled
1 (15-ounce) can kidney, navy,
or garbanzo beans
½ cup grated Parmesan
cheese
1 cup fresh basil leaves,
minced

You can use any pasta for this recipe, but rotini is the
best at holding on to vegetables and dressing. For fun,
look for green, red, or multicolored pasta.

1. In a large bowl whisk together vinegar, garlic, Italian seasoning, and oil.

2. Add onion, tomatoes, bell pepper, pasta, and beans and toss to coat.

3. Cover and chill 1 hour or overnight to allow flavors to mingle.

4. Pack in a plastic container and top with Parmesan and basil.

Mom's Trail Mix

The beauty of this mix is that it can be tailored to your family's taste. If you have a thing for dried apricots, toss them in. Prefer cashews to peanuts? Switch it up. Want to add a teaspoon of flax? Go right ahead. It's your mix.

Combine all ingredients in a large bowl and mix well. Store in an airtight container, and pack in plastic zipper bags for easy transport.

7 CUPS OF SNACK MIX, ENOUGH FOR A WEEK OF NIBBLING

per 1 cup of trail mix
580 calories
35 g fat
56 g carbohydrates
17 g protein
90 mg sodium
9 g fiber

INGREDIENTS
1 cup peanuts
1 cup almonds
1 cup golden raisins
1 cup sunflower seeds, hulled
2 cups low-fat granola
1 cup shredded coconut

Ants, Ladybugs, and Crickets on Logs

To transport these sticky snacks, stack two celery sticks together, sticky sides touching, before wrapping them up in wax paper.

1. Fill half of the celery sticks with peanut butter and half with cream cheese.

2. Top with raisins, cranberries, and nuts in assorted combinations, and serve.

SERVES 8

190 calories
15 g fat
12 g carbohydrates
6 g protein
150 mg sodium
2 g fiber

INGREDIENTS
6 stalks celery, washed, trimmed, and cut into 3-inch lengths
½ cup peanut butter
½ cup cream cheese
¼ cup raisins
¼ cup dried cranberries
¼ cup sliced almonds

Cheesy Popcorn

Popcorn is fun. But more importantly, it's full of fiber and fulfills a serving of whole grain. Parmesan cheese is salty, but not too fatty. Plus, it has calcium. Munch away!

Pop corn in an air popper or microwave. While hot, top with cheese and serve.

Micropop

To pop in a microwave, place corn in a paper bag, seal it tightly, and heat for about 2 minutes on high. Be careful opening the bag, as it will be full of hot steam.

SERVES 2

120 calories
3 g fat
18 g carbohydrates
5 g protein
95 mg sodium
3 g fiber

INGREDIENTS
¼ cup popcorn
2–3 tablespoons grated
    Parmesan cheese

Fruit Kebabs

The best fruit kebabs are made with fresh, seasonal fruit. Try bananas, pineapples, melon, berries, peaches, grapes, and mango. If your pickings are slim, use canned or frozen fruit, but not if it is packed in sugar syrup.

Thread fruit on skewers in an alternating pattern. Serve with yogurt for dipping.

SERVES 4

180 calories
1 g fat
43 g carbohydrates
5 g protein
50 mg sodium
4 g fiber

INGREDIENTS
6–8 cups assorted seasonal
    fruits, cut into 1-inch
    chunks
6–8 wooden skewers
1 cup plain nonfat yogurt

Chapter 16

Cooking with the Kids

Cooking at home is the very best way to stay healthy, and to bring your family together. As soon as your kids can walk, it's time to get them involved. Toddlers can be a part of the action by coloring placemats or name cards and helping someone older set the table. But once they reach elementary school, it's time to get them cooking. This chapter includes great information, tips, and recipes for cooking with your kids at home.

Beyond Pizza and Cookies

Kids should be familiar with all parts of the kitchen, and be able to feed themselves without fear of burning the house down. It's also important to show them that there is more to mealtime than setting, clearing, and washing the dishes. The best way to make that happen is to start them early.

Most cooking courses for kids teach "kid food," like pizza and cookies. It's fun for them, but it does not teach them how to really cook for themselves. These courses concentrate on recipes, and ignore personal taste. When a parent does the teaching, the lessons are tailored to the student, and the mini chef will be better able to explore his own creativity in the kitchen, which is where all the fun is.

An easy place to start your cooking lessons is at breakfast. Breakfast meals are usually fairly simple to prepare, they have few ingredients, and they can be enjoyed right away. Cereal is a no-brainer, but there are still things to learn, such as serving the correct portion, pouring milk without spilling, and the proper way to clean up spilt milk. Don't forget to show the proper way to store food to keep it fresh.

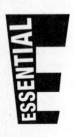

For more complex lessons, like toast, eggs, or oatmeal, be sure to allot enough time in the morning to assist. The first few lessons might be best learned on a weekend, when stress to get out the door doesn't overshadow the joy of cooking. Then, after a few Saturdays, try it on a school day.

Lunch, too, is another good starting point. Sandwiches are simple, but cutting up fruit and vegetables may take some training, not to mention packing things properly to keep them fresh and spill-proof. In the winter months, a batch of homemade soup in a thermos will be the envy of the playground. Kids are much more likely to eat a lunch they pack themselves.

Dinnertime is family time, and it is a great time to get everyone together. Basic helping skills will grow into preparation of a course, and eventually an entire meal. While holidays and special events often see families cooking together, making it an everyday event prolongs the daily together time and provides an opportunity not just for culinary training, but also for broader "quality-time" discussions.

Techniques to Emphasize

When teaching cooking to kids or adults, there are basic skills that must be addressed. First and foremost is safety and sanitation.

Safety First

Children should be able to navigate the kitchen safely. Show them everything that gets hot, including the hot tap of the sink. Describe how the stove works, and teach them to turn it on and off. If you have a gas range, point out the pilot light and explain the mechanism. If yours is electric, spend time watching the coils heat and turn red. Do the same with the oven, toaster, and any other countertop appliance that little fingers can get stuck in. If they learn what the appliances are for, and how to operate them, they are less likely to experiment with them on the sly. Don't forget to give rules for the microwave, including no metal or tin foil.

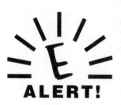

Knives in the sink water can get hidden under the soapy bubbles. Blindly reaching in to do the dishes can result in a nasty cut. Leave them on the edge of the sink.

Reveal where the sharp knives are kept, and demonstrate how to use them properly. Show the wrong way, too. Cut something, and explain that the blade cuts everything that way, even fingers. Explain knife safety rules, such as no walking or running around with a knife. Put it down on the counter, don't drop it into the sink water, don't point it at anyone, and never, ever play with it.

Keep It Clean

Keep hair tied back, wear short sleeves, and give everyone an apron. Discuss sanitation and germs. Talk about food on clothing and how it can spread germs to other places and people in the house. Show the proper way to wash hands before handling food and explain when hands need to be rewashed.

Talk about cross-contamination and how one should always use a separate cutting board for meat. Show how to clean as you cook, keeping work areas tidy and keeping up with dirty dishes. Explain that the floor is not a garbage can, and that someone (usually the messiest one) needs to sweep it after the cooking is complete.

Teacher Training

There is no curriculum to follow when teaching your kids to cook. There is only opportunity and encouragement. Try to be patient, and let them make messes and mistakes. Many of the best lessons are learned from mistakes. If you constantly finish things for them, they will not learn, and the experience will be less interesting for them.

Not all kids show an interest in cooking, which is fine. Not everyone has to love it. Everyone does need to learn basic skills to feed themselves, and to pull their weight with the family chores. For these kids, keep the lessons as short and as delicious as you can.

Teaching the Food Label

When teaching kids to cook, it is especially important to show them healthy ingredients. Discuss with them the recommended dietary guidelines discussed in Chapter 2. At the market, point out the different choices, and discuss which option would be the healthiest. The food label is on practically everything, so there is ample opportunity to compare. In your kitchen, show them where to find the label and discuss its different components. Specifically show them the sugar, fiber, protein, and fat listings. Even younger kids should be able to look at the label and find these basic nutrients. (Read about the food label in Chapter 3.)

You can really empower older kids by diving a little deeper into the contents of their food.

Pick a food you know to be high in fat and show its food label. Discuss fat, our need for it, and our overuse of it. Do the same with fiber, sugar, protein, and sodium. Then, take them to the market and let them pick the best products for you.

Supermarket Scavenger Hunt

The following activity is designed to get your kids reading labels and make them aware of what is in the foods they eat. Give them these questions, a clipboard, a pencil, and let them loose in the supermarket. (It's best to do this during a slow shopping time.) It will take about an hour to complete, so you may want to divide it up into a few smaller trips. When they have completed the hunt, discuss their findings. It will be an eye-opening experience for them.

1. **Find a low-fat or low-calorie ice cream.**
   - Name of product:
   - Serving size:
   - Calories per serving:
   - Percent of fat per serving:
   - Does it contain hydrogenated fat?
2. **Find the fat percentage in a single serving of the following items:**
   - Hot dog
   - Veggie dog
   - Plain yogurt
   - Low-fat plain yogurt
   - Italian salad dressing
   - Ranch salad dressing
   - Cheddar cheese
   - Low-fat Cheddar cheese
   - Which product had the most fat? Which had the least?
3. **Find the calories per serving of the following items:**
   - Strawberry jam
   - Sugar-free strawberry jam

- Whole milk
- Fat-free milk
- Sour cream
- Low-fat sour cream
- Which products have the most calories? Which have the least?

4. **Pick your favorite cookie and find out:**
   - Name of product:
   - Serving size:
   - Calories per serving:
   - Percent of sugar per serving:
   - Does it contain hydrogenated fat?
   - How many different types of sugar can you find in the ingredients? (Hint: their names end in "ose")

5. **Find a cookie with the least amount of calories.**
   - Name of product:
   - Serving size:
   - Calories per serving:
   - Percent of sugar per serving:
   - Does it contain hydrogenated fat?

6. **Find the sodium per serving of the following products:**
   - Ketchup
   - Mustard
   - Chicken noodle soup
   - Ramen
   - Potato chips
   - Pretzels
   - Are there low-sodium versions of the same products?

7. **Find four cereals with at least four grams of fiber per serving.**
   - Name of product:
   - Serving size:
   - Grams of fiber per serving:
   - Name of product:
   - Serving size:
   - Grams of fiber per serving:
   - Name of product:
   - Serving size:

- Grams of fiber per serving:
- Name of product:
- Serving size:
- · Grams of fiber per serving:

8. **Find a loaf of white bread and find out:**
   - Name of product:
   - Calories per slice:
   - Grams of fiber per slice:
   - First ingredient listed:

9. **Find a loaf of multigrain bread (seven-grain, twelve-grain, etc.) and find out:**
   - Name of product:
   - Calories per slice:
   - Grams of fiber per slice:
   - First ingredient listed:

10. **Find the percentage of sugar per serving in the following products:**
    - Cola
    - Ketchup
    - Fat-free ranch dressing
    - Ice cream sandwiches
    - Jell-O
    - Which product had the most sugar? Which had the least?

You can extend the scavenger hunt idea into many different arenas. Try a hunt for fruits and vegetables. A simple list will get them reading signs and identifying produce.

Family Menu Planning

Showing kids how to plan a menu is great experience and an important skill to learn. The ability to organize and plan can be applied to all aspects of their lives, from cleaning their rooms and doing homework to college and their own household management.

The first step in menu planning is to make a list. List the meals and snacks for an entire week. Be sure to give the kids a say in the food they make and eat. (Of course, parents have veto power.) A useful strategy includes giving every family member a day of the week to have their favorite meal.

Organize the meals and snacks in a calendar form, then take a good look at it. How does the week's menu compare to dietary guidelines? It may take a bit of adjusting before it meets them. Remember to serve a majority of whole-grain foods at every meal, lots of vegetables, and about two servings of protein a day. Limit fat and sugar, and opt for fruit as a sweet treat, rather than cookies or ice cream, at least on a daily basis.

Print the menu out and post it on the fridge. Let the kids decorate it for the season. Use the menu to create your shopping list. By repeating the menu for several weeks you can save money buying products in larger quantities. At the market, you can divide up the list and send the kids off in a hunt for the things you need. Change the menu once in a while, to keep everyone from getting bored.

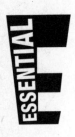

Shopping provides an opportunity to teach kids about price and value. Show them the different brands and compare prices. Is there something on sale? Do you have coupons? Is the quantity in each brand the same? How is it packaged? All these elements play a role in determining the best value.

Now everyone has proudly participated in meal preparation. As they grow older, having taken part in this process will make them better able to handle it on their own.

Easy, Healthy Recipes for Young Cooks

The following recipes teach real cooking skills and will add real, healthy recipes to your weekly menu.

Whole-Wheat Banana-Nut Pancakes

For a superior banana-nut pancake, use bananas that are nearly overripe. If it's cold out, don't forget to warm the syrup on the stove or in the microwave.

1. In a medium-size bowl sift together flour, baking powder, and salt.

2. In a separate bowl, combine milk, oil, honey, and eggs. Whisk together thoroughly.

3. Pour the egg mixture into the sifted dry ingredients, along with the nuts and bananas, and stir to combine. Be careful not to overmix. A few lumps are okay. Set aside at room temperature for 10 minutes.

4. Heat griddle over high heat and oil it lightly. Test the griddle by sprin- g on a little water. If it sizzles and evaporates, it's ready.

5. Lower the heat to medium and ladle out the batter. Cook for 1–2 minutes, until bubbles appear.

6. Flip the pancake and cook the other side, about 1–2 minutes. Adjust the heat of your griddle as necessary.

7. Repeat with remaining batter. Serve immediately, or keep warm in a 200°F oven, covered with foil.

SERVES 4

610 calories
33 g fat
69 g carbohydrates
18 g protein
680 mg sodium
9 g fiber

INGREDIENTS
1½ cups whole-wheat flour
2½ teaspoons baking powder
½ teaspoon kosher salt
1½ cups fat-free milk
3 tablespoons peanut oil
3 tablespoons honey
2 eggs
1 cup toasted walnuts
2 bananas, sliced

Gazpacho

SERVES 6

250 calories
19 g fat
19 g carbohydrates
5 g protein
1,050 mg sodium
4 g fiber

INGREDIENTS

*2 dinner rolls, soaked in
1 cup of water for 10
minutes*
6 ripe tomatoes, chopped
*1 cup cucumber, peeled,
seeded, and chopped*
*1 cup red bell pepper,
chopped*
3 scallions, chopped
2 cloves garlic, chopped
*2 tablespoons red wine
vinegar*
½ cup olive oil
½ tablespoon kosher salt
*1–2 tablespoons ground
cumin*
*1–2 tablespoons hot pepper
sauce (to your liking)*
2–4 cups tomato juice
½ cup nonfat plain yogurt

*This soup is refreshing on hot summer days. Make sure you use
fresh, high-quality veggies for this soup.*

1. In a large bowl, combine all ingredients, mix well, and refrigerate for 1
   hour or overnight to mingle flavors.

2. Working in batches, puree in a blender to desired consistency.

3. Serve chilled, with a dollop of nonfat plain yogurt.

Croque Monsieur

Croque Monsieur (pronounced "croak-miss-ur") means Mister Crunchy. In France these grilled cheese sandwiches can be found on every street corner. There, they contain Gruyere cheese, a wee bit of ham, and sometimes a little béchamel sauce. A Croque Madam is the same sandwich, with a fried egg added into the mix. If you'd like to add the ham or egg, do so in the center of the cheese.

1. Brush each slice of bread with olive oil.

2. Lay one slice in a nonstick skillet, oil side down.

3. Put the cheese on top and cover it with the second slice of bread, oil side up.

4. Place the pan over medium heat and cook until the bottom is golden brown, about 2 minutes.

5. Carefully flip sandwich over and brown the other side. Cut the sandwich on the diagonal and serve.

Careful, Please!

When using a nonstick pan, be sure to use a heat-resistant plastic spatula. Flipping food in a nonstick pan with a metal tool scrapes off the nonstick surface.

SERVES 2

580 calories
44 g fat
29 g carbohydrates
20 g protein
400 mg sodium
4 g fiber

INGREDIENTS
*4 slices whole-wheat
     sandwich bread
4 tablespoons olive oil
1 cup grated Swiss cheese*

Vegetable Lasagna

There is no need to preboil the noodles for lasagna. There is enough moisture and heat in the center of the lasagna to cook the noodles in the oven. If you'd like to make this a meaty lasagna, add a half pound of ground turkey or lean beef with the sautéed onions.

1. Preheat oven to 350°F.

2. In a large sauce pan, sauté onion and garlic in olive oil until tender.

3. Add oregano, basil, fennel seed, sage, mushrooms, and zucchini, and continue to cook until tender and dry.

4. Add artichokes and tomato sauce, reduce heat, and simmer for 10–15 minutes to warm through.

5. Cover the bottom of the lasagna pan with a thin layer of sauce to prevent the noodles from burning. Lay three lasagna noodles in the bottom of the pan, being careful not to overlap too much. Break them into pieces if necessary to cover the bottom of the pan.

6. Add ¼ inch of sauce, a generous handful of grated mozzarella, a layer of spinach leaves, and 4–5 dollops of ricotta cheese. Cover with another layer of noodles as before, and repeat layering.

7. Finish the layering with sauce, mozzarella, and Parmesan cheese.

8. Cover and bake until the sauce is bubbly and the cheese is melted, about 30 minutes. Uncover the dish and cook another 10 minutes to brown the top. Serve hot.

SERVES 4–6

820 calories
32 g fat
89 g carbohydrates
49 g protein
1,480 mg sodium
11 g fiber

INGREDIENTS
2–4 tablespoons olive oil
1 large yellow onion, diced
6 large cloves of garlic, minced
3 tablespoons dried oregano
2 tablespoons dried basil
1 tablespoon dried crushed fennel seed
1 tablespoon dried sage
8 ounces chopped mushrooms
1 large zucchini, grated
1 (15-ounce) can artichokes, chopped
1 (29-ounce) can tomato sauce
1 (1-pound) package lasagna noodles
1 (15-ounce) package part-skim ricotta cheese (optional)
4 cups fresh spinach leaves
1 pound low-moisture, part-skim mozzarella cheese, grated, divided into 4 portions
½ cup Parmesan cheese, grated

Recipes to Introduce International Flavors to Kids

The next recipes are designed to open their minds and awaken their taste buds.

Baba Ghanoush

*Like hummus, baba ghanoush is a staple in the Middle East.
Serve it with pita bread, or Pita Chips (page 208).*

1. Preheat oven to 400°F.

2. Coat eggplant and garlic lightly with olive oil, place on a baking sheet, and roast until brown and soft, 30–40 minutes.

3. Cool and peel the eggplant and put it in a food processor.

4. Cut garlic in half, squeeze out the soft roasted cloves, and put in the processor.

5. Add remaining ingredients and puree, adding enough olive oil to reach a smooth, yogurt-like consistency.

6. Transfer to serving bowl and swirl the top with a spoon.

7. Drizzle on a generous amount of olive oil and sprinkle liberally with chopped parsley and/or ground paprika.

SERVES 6

220 calories
15 g fat
20 g carbohydrates
5 g protein
200 mg sodium
7 g fiber

INGREDIENTS
2 large eggplants
2 bulbs garlic
1 medium yellow onion, chopped
¼ cup tahini
¼ cup lemon juice
½ teaspoon kosher salt
½ teaspoon ground black pepper
¼–½ cup olive oil

Pita Chips

These chips are great for dipping, but they also stand alone as a terrific snack. They are a healthy, and surprisingly popular, alternative to potato chips. You can also make a sweet version by replacing the savory spices and oil with cinnamon and honey. Watch them carefully in the oven. The bread is very thin, and they can burn easily. It may require a little stirring to ensure even browning.

SERVES 8

310 calories
17 g fat
36 g carbohydrates
8 g protein
430 mg sodium
5 g fiber

INGREDIENTS

8 pita pocket bread rounds
½ cup olive oil
2 cloves garlic, minced
½ teaspoon dried oregano
½ teaspoon dried basil
½ teaspoon dried rosemary
½ teaspoon black pepper
½ cup Parmesan cheese

1. In a small bowl combine olive oil, garlic, oregano, basil, rosemary, and black pepper. Stir to combine and set aside to infuse flavors, at least 30 minutes, or overnight.

2. Preheat oven to 400°F. Coat 2–3 baking sheets with pan spray.

3. Cut each pita round into eight triangles, separate halves, and spread on baking sheets in a single layer.

4. Brush oil mixture lightly onto each pita triangle. Sprinkle with Parmesan cheese.

5. Bake 5–7 minutes, until golden brown and crisp.

Chicken Madras

Madras is the former name of the fourth-largest city in India, now called Chennai, on the country's southeastern coast. If you buy traditional madras sauce or powder, you'll find it red and full of spicy chilies. Yellow curry, or garam masala, is generally milder.

1. Heat oil in a large sauté pan over high heat, and sauté onion until tender.

2. Mix together chicken, curry, lemon juice, and salt. Add to sauté pan and brown, 3–5 minutes.

3. Add potatoes, raisins, and enough water to cover.

4. Reduce heat, cover, and simmer 20 minutes, until potatoes are tender.

5. Just before serving, stir in cilantro. Serve with brown rice and nonfat plain yogurt.

SERVES 4

280 calories
9 g fat
34 g carbohydrates
15 g protein
325 mg sodium
4 g fiber

INGREDIENTS

2 tablespoons olive oil
1 large onion, diced
2 skinless, boneless chicken breasts
2–4 tablespoons garam masala
¼ cup lemon juice
1 teaspoon kosher salt
6 new potatoes, halved
½ cup golden raisins
2–4 cups water
1 cup fresh cilantro, chopped

Thai Coconut Soup

SERVES 4

280 calories
13 g fat
6 g carbohydrates
34 g protein
1,450 mg sodium
3 g fiber

INGREDIENTS
1 (5.6-ounce) can coconut
    milk
4 cups chicken broth
¼ cup fresh ginger, grated
2 tablespoons grated lemon
    zest
2 tablespoons grated lime
    zest
4 tablespoons fish sauce
1 tablespoon red chili flakes
3 cups cooked chicken,
    shredded
¼ cup fresh cilantro, chopped

In Thailand the name of this soup is Thom Kha Gai. *The flavor combination of lime, coconut, and ginger is heavenly.*

1. In a large soup pot, combine coconut milk, chicken broth, ginger, lemon zest, and lime zest. Bring to a boil, reduce heat, and simmer 30 minutes. Strain and return liquid to the pot.

2. Add fish sauce, chili flakes, and chicken. Simmer 30 minutes more. Serve hot with lime wedges and chopped cilantro.

Nam Pla
Fish sauce, also called nam pla *in Thailand, is an ancient condiment well loved by the Romans, who called it* garum. *They produced it throughout the ancient Mediterranean region. Today, you can find it wherever Asian groceries are sold.*

Raspberry Crepes

Crepes can be filled with anything, sweet or savory. They can also be made well ahead of time and stored in the fridge for a day or two, or in the freezer for a week. To serve, simply warm them up briefly in a dry nonstick pan.

1. Combine eggs, flour, milk, water, and salt in a blender and mix to the consistency of thin cream. Refrigerate 1–3 hours.

2. Heat a nonstick pan over high heat. Add a little butter, let it sizzle, then add enough batter to thinly coat the bottom of the pan. Cook, swirling the pan, for 1 minute. Flip and cook the other side another minute, until golden brown. Turn out onto a plate, and repeat with remaining batter. (It is usually not necessary to butter the pan more than once.)

3. In a small sauce pan, combine berries, jam, and honey, and cook until heated through.

4. Place a tablespoon of fruit in the center of each crepe, fold into quarters, and serve immediately.

SERVES 4

140 calories
4 g fat
22 g carbohydrates
6 g protein
200 mg sodium
4 g fiber

INGREDIENTS
1–2 tablespoons butter, as needed
3 eggs
2 tablespoons whole-wheat flour
1 tablespoon nonfat milk
1 tablespoon water
¼ teaspoon kosher salt
1 pint raspberries
2 tablespoons sugar-free raspberry jam
2 tablespoons honey

Chapter 17

Nutrition for Teenagers and College Kids

Older kids are a lot more mobile, and a lot less visible, than little ones. Soon enough, you'll have to let go, and have faith that you've taught them well. Their teenage years, sixth through twelfth grade, are your final chance to instill a healthy mindset. Teenagers grow rapidly. You will see a noticeable increase in physical size as well as a greater need for sleep—and the inevitable mood swings. Good nutrition is vital to this stage of growth, but it is all too often overlooked because kids are spending more time away from home and are more responsible for feeding themselves.

Damage Control

The difficulty in this age bracket is that children are surrounded by temptation. Availability of junk food is widespread. Even school lunchtime offerings are full of empty, mind-numbing calories. After school the need to placate kids with snacks is universal. Snacktime culture exists everywhere, from friends' houses to scout meetings, at team practice and music lessons. Kids need to know what these foods do to them and they need viable alternatives.

If up until this point you have encouraged a healthy diet, your children may need only to be reminded of the basics. The main culprits are sugar and fat. Remind them of the effects sugar has on their performance in all aspects of life. The sugar crash is a terrible thing when it happens in algebra class.

Combat Advertising

There are lots of reasons to limit your kids' television time, many of which have no bearing on health or nutrition. But besides the obvious need to get them off the couch and moving around, limiting television can make your job as nutrition monitor much easier. Less television means fewer advertisements, and that directly reduces the number of products your kids will want to try. Do not underestimate the power of these ads. Kids will flatly turn down products that are not the right brand.

Try the following exercise to make television viewing a learning experience. Have the kids write down each product advertised and ask them about the ad itself. Who is it targeting? What is it using to draw the attention of these groups? What benefits does the ad claim to provide? When kids consider these aspects of advertising, they can see the medium in a new light and become cautious, skeptical consumers.

Take the information gathered from the ads to the store and investigate the products first-hand. Read the labels and compare nutrients. Look at the packaging and talk about the target audience. See if you can find similar products with a different target. Giving them the tools to filter out the peripheral information and dig down to the essentials is another skill that will serve them well throughout life.

Hormones and Food

The onslaught of hormones and the stress of a growing body coupled with increased peer pressure make this a tough time of life. But believe it or not, good nutrition can help ease much of the discomfort of adolescent limbo.

Kids in this age bracket are growing rapidly. They need more calories and an increase of certain nutrients to meet these growth demands. The average teenager needs 2,500–3,000 calories a day, and more if they are physically active on a daily basis. You may notice your teenager eating like a horse and still not feeling satisfied. As long as the meals are healthful, there is no cause for concern. If these meals originate at the drive-through, then problems can arise.

Poor eating habits at this age frequently lead to reduced intake of calcium and iron. Teenagers must go through growth spurts, just as they did when they were little. Bones are not yet fully developed, and calcium is still a very necessary component of their everyday diet. They need two to three servings of low-fat or fat-free dairy products each day. This form of calcium is the easiest form for their bodies to absorb.

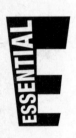

Teenage nutrition can be challenging, but if the kids understand what is at stake, you may find they have a positive attitude. Remind them that good nutrition can help them reach their goals. It enhances athletic ability; produces healthy-looking hair, skin, and teeth; and optimizes the development of muscle.

Growth spurts will also lead to an increased need for rest. But excessive fatigue can be a signal of anemia, so it is important to monitor their iron intake.

Adequate protein is important for growing bodies. Teenagers need from forty-four to sixty grams of protein a day, which is usually not hard to get. Unfortunately, often excessively fatty protein is what kids choose. Make lean protein available to them.

Vitamins are especially important now, and the more they get from natural sources, the better. Thiamin, riboflavin, and niacin are crucial to help release energy from increased consumption of carbohydrates. Vitamin B_6, vitamin B_{12}, and folate are needed to support increased muscle mass and expanded blood supply. Vitamin D helps strengthen bones through growth spurts, and vitamins A, C, and E help protect all the newly formed cells.

Positive Food Relationships

During the teen years, boys and girls become increasingly different. By the time they are through growing, boys will double their muscle mass, and girls will gain more body fat. Normal body fat for teenagers is 12 percent for boys, and 23 percent for girls. You can estimate body fat by calculating your body mass index (BMI). You can read about BMI in Chapter 20.

As kids enter adolescence, their growth rates vary dramatically. Girls typically gain weight a full six to nine months before they start getting taller. Estrogen and progesterone promote the deposit of abdominal fat, a widened pelvis, and broadened hips. Boys gain both height and weight simultaneously, usually a little later than the girls. Testosterone increases muscle mass and strengthens bones. All of this happens to every single teenager, and yet, in their self-absorbed adolescent world, they think they are going it alone. This is the time to emphasize a positive body image.

There is no way to block the assault on teens' body image. It comes at them from every direction. Television, movies, books, magazines, music, and their peers are all dictating what is pretty and cool, and what is not. It takes real fortitude to foster a good self-image in the midst of all this.

If up until now nutrition has been a family focus, and the relationship with food is healthy, there is little cause for alarm. But even a healthy kid can experience poor body image. Teenagers can easily adopt unrealistic ideas regarding their appearance. Because of this, parents should pay attention to food consumption, and food relationships.

Parents should encourage the use of healthy dietary guidelines and discourage fad diets. They should also encourage exercise, but not excessive exercise. Watch your kids and their relationship to food and dieting. If they seem overly interested in dieting or weight loss, especially if they are at a normal, healthy weight, take some time to discuss these issues with them. If they seem withdrawn or they want to eat alone, there is cause for concern about an eating disorder. Hiding weight loss under loose clothing, skipping meals, and cutting out certain foods are further indications. Consult the family doctor if you suspect an eating disorder.

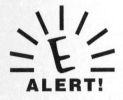

Remember to emphasize that food is fuel and not a substitute for friendship. It is common to view food as a comfort item, but excessive fat and sugar is no less damaging simply because you're depressed.

Developing Culinary Skills

Getting kids to help around the kitchen in the early years is a great start to self-reliance. This trend must continue through the teen years if kids are going to make a successful go of it on their own. Assuming you have already covered the basics, it's time to up the ante.

Encourage your teens to try new recipes. Introducing them to foreign foods is a great way to start this. Center a meal around a particular country and have everyone in the family contribute a dish to the table. Or have the kids orchestrate an entire meal without the help of the parents.

You can also get them to include their friends in their culinary exploits. Have them form a dinner club in which each member takes turns cooking a meal around a specific theme. It could be a country, movie, era, or season. Anything goes. Kids can dress the part too, and make it a real social event.

Healthy Decision Making

When your children finally leave the nest, all you can do is hope for the best. If it is college life they're heading off to, take some time to review nutrition and healthy habits. Campus life is brutal to good nutrition, but the lessons learned throughout childhood and adolescence can carry them through relatively unscathed.

Once again, emphasis on food as fuel can make the point. A balanced diet will provide increased stamina for late-night studying and long-winded lectures. And a healthy diet will help them bounce back after the inevitable parties. If you focus on the goal, the road to it can seem less daunting.

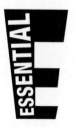

Why not suggest a homemade meal as their gift for Mother's or Father's Day, an anniversary, or a birthday? It will be cheaper for them, and more meaningful than another necktie or bottle of perfume.

The Freshman Ten

On many campuses, the cost of meals at the cafeteria is included in the tuition. That means there is a never-ending supply of macaroni and cheese, and soft-serve ice cream. The temptation is too much for most kids, which is why they have a name for the poundage gained in the first year away from home.

This phenomenon is not limited to college life, however. The first time kids are left to fend for themselves, without restrictions or visible consequences, they will, like monkeys caged for eighteen years, go wild. But if you have trained them right, it will only take a few mornings of heartburn, or worse, to remind them of their need for healthy, balanced fuel.

One way to help arm them against the free-for-all frenzy of the young single life is with some really good recipes. The ones in this chapter will provide them with an alternative to late-night fast food and also save them money. In addition they will definitely impress their friends. What more could they want?

Easy, Healthy Recipes for Beginner Cooks

The following recipes are easy, delicious, and very mature.

Crudités with Creamy Herb Dip

SERVES 8

90 calories
4 g fat
7 g carbohydrates
9 g protein
410 mg sodium
2 g fiber

INGREDIENTS

2 cups cottage cheese
½ cup sour cream
4 green onions, minced
2 tablespoons fresh chives,
  minced
2 tablespoons fresh parsley,
  minced
1 tablespoon fresh dill,
  minced
½ teaspoon kosher salt
½ teaspoon black pepper
½ teaspoon onion powder
1 large purple cabbage
5–6 cups assorted
  vegetables, peeled and
  chopped

The great thing about this recipe is that you can use whatever vegetables you like, and whatever looks good in the market. Carrot and celery sticks are easy, as are cucumber wheels and cherry tomatoes. Or try broccoli and cauliflower florets, snap peas, bell peppers, or jicama.

1. In a blender, combine cottage cheese and sour cream and blend until smooth.

2. Transfer to a large bowl and add onions, chives, parsley, dill, salt, pepper, and onion powder. Blend well, cover and chill for at least 1 hour, or overnight to mingle flavors.

3. Carefully remove the large outer leaves of a purple cabbage, reshape them into a bowl, and fill with the herbed dip. Set cabbage bowl in the center of a platter and arrange cut vegetables all around. Serve chilled.

Caprese Salad

The name of this salad in Italian is Insalata Caprese, *which means "salad in the style of Capri." Capri is an island in the Bay of Naples, in the region of Campania. The colors of this salad are said to represent the colors of the Italian flag.*

On each serving plate arrange alternately slices of tomato, mozzarella, and basil leaves. Drizzle with olive oil, sprinkle with salt and pepper, and serve.

Buffalo Cheese?

Mozzarella di Bufala Campana is fresh (not aged) cheese made from the milk of water buffalos. It is exported to the United States and copied by several cheese manufacturers. Fresh mozzarella is sold floating in mild brine, and should be consumed within two days of purchase.

SERVES 4

320 calories
27 g fat
8 g carbohydrates
12 g protein
380 mg sodium
3 g fiber

INGREDIENTS

2 ripe tomatoes, sliced thinly
8 ounces buffalo mozzarella, sliced thinly
1 cup large fresh basil leaves
¼ cup extra virgin olive oil
½ teaspoon sea or kosher salt
½ teaspoon freshly cracked black pepper

Mixed Green Salad with Herb Vinaigrette

SERVES 4

70 calories
7 g fat
3 g carbohydrates
1 g protein
350 mg sodium
1 g fiber

INGREDIENTS

*Juice and zest of 1 lemon
  (about 2 tablespoons)
½ teaspoon kosher salt
½ teaspoon ground black
  pepper
1 tablespoon Dijon mustard
1–2 tablespoons fresh chives,
  chopped
1–2 tablespoons fresh parsley,
  chopped
1–2 tablespoons fresh basil,
  chopped
1–2 tablespoons fresh
  tarragon
2 tablespoons olive oil
4 cups mixed greens*

Mixed salad greens are available in most markets premixed, pre-cut, prewashed, and sealed in bags. But beware. These bagged greens spoil quickly once opened. Buy only what you need, and if you can, buy loose mixed greens.

In a large bowl, whisk together lemon juice and zest, salt, pepper, mustard, and fresh herbs. Slowly drizzle in oil while whisking. Add greens, toss to coat, and serve immediately.

Chicken Stir-Fry

The key to this recipe is cooking over very high heat. Woks are designed to hold the heat and transfer it evenly throughout the pan. If you don't have a wok, a good sauté pan is a pretty good substitute. Be sure to keep the food moving as it cooks.

1. In a large bowl combine chicken, cornstarch, ginger, soy sauce, sesame oil, honey, and rice vinegar. Mix well and marinate at least 1 hour, or overnight.

2. In a wok or sauté pan over high heat, remove chicken from marinade and cook in peanut oil, stirring, until done, about 3–4 minutes. Reserve marinade. Remove chicken from pan and set aside.

3. To the hot pan add celery, carrots, peas, bean sprouts, and cashews and cook until browned.

4. Return chicken to pan, add marinade, and bring to boil. Cook until thick, about 5 minutes. Serve over brown rice, topped with green onions.

Ginger Root

Fresh ginger root is available in most supermarkets. Grate it, using the finest holes on your grater, until you reach the fibrous center. Two teaspoons of ground ginger can be substituted in this recipe.

SERVES 4–6

430 calories
26 g fat
31 g carbohydrates
22 g protein
1,090 mg sodium
4 g fiber

INGREDIENTS
2 boneless, skinless chicken breasts, cut in strips
2 tablespoons cornstarch
2 tablespoons fresh grated ginger
¼ cup soy sauce
2 tablespoons sesame oil
2 tablespoons honey
½ cup rice vinegar
3 tablespoons peanut oil
2 stalks celery, slices
1 carrot, sliced
1 cup snow peas
1 cup bean sprouts
½ cup cashews, chopped
½ cup green onions

Foil-Baked Salmon

SERVES 4

250 calories
16 g fat
10 g carbohydrates
20 g protein
60 mg sodium
3 g fiber

INGREDIENTS

4 (3-ounce) salmon filets
3 tablespoons olive oil
½ teaspoon black pepper
1 cup green onions, chopped
2 tablespoons fresh dill,
  minced
1 cup baby carrots, sliced
1 bunch asparagus, sliced 1
  inch wide
1 cup zucchini, sliced
Juice of 1 lemon

This is a modern version of the French method en papillote, *which means "in paper." Wrapped in parchment paper, the moisture of the food is trapped, and the steam cooks the food. It has an added benefit of trapping all the flavor, aroma, and nutrients.*

1. Preheat oven to 400°F.

2. Place each piece of salmon on a large sheet of foil, brushed lightly with oil. Brush fish with oil, sprinkle with pepper and dill. Divide onions, carrots, asparagus, and zucchini evenly between each filet, and place on top. Sprinkle with a squeeze of lemon juice.

3. Wrap foil up and over fish, and fold to seal tightly. Place on a baking sheet and bake for 15–20 minutes, until the fish is firm and cooked through. (Cooking time is approximately 10 minutes per inch of fish, so remember to measure the thickness before you wrap it up.)

Safe Salmon

Much of the salmon available in markets today is farmed, or aquacultured. While salmon is high in the heart-healthy omego-3 fatty acids, recent studies indicate that toxin levels in aquacultured salmon is ten times higher than that of wild salmon. Toxins are thought to originate in the feed, which is made from fish caught in polluted waters. So look for wild salmon, and limit your intake of farmed salmon to once or twice a month.

Pasta Primavera

This is a simple dish, but it can be easily ruined by overcooking. To get it right, cut the vegetables as uniformly in size as possible, blanch to the proper doneness, then chill and hold them until the pasta is ready. The goal is to keep these vegetables vibrant in color, texture, and flavor.

1. Fill a large pasta pot with water and bring to a rolling boil. Add vegetables, one type at a time, and cook 3–5 minutes, until tender but still bright. Transfer immediately to ice water.

2. Fill pot with water again and bring to a rolling boil. At the boil, add pasta and cook al dente. Drain, rinse with cold water, and toss with 1 tablespoon olive oil.

3. Heat remaining oil in large sauté pan over high heat. Add shallots and cook until tender.

4. Add cream, parsley, and basil, and bring to boil.

5. Add blanched vegetables, pasta, tomatoes, salt, pepper, and Parmesan cheese. Toss to coat, and serve immediately.

Pasta Perfect

Let your pasta shape determine the size of your vegetables. The vegetables should be no larger than the pasta. Linguini or fettuccini are long and thin, so their vegetables should be in julienne strips. Shell or bowtie pasta should be accompanied by small or medium diced veggies.

SERVES 6

470 calories
15 g fat
69 g carbohydrates
17 g protein
190 mg sodium
5 g fiber

INGREDIENTS
8 baby carrots
8 baby zucchini
8 baby yellow squash
1 red bell pepper
8 spears asparagus
1 cup baby peas
1 pound fettuccini
3 tablespoons olive oil
2 shallots, minced
1 cup half-and-half
¼ cup fresh flat leaf parsley
¼ cup fresh basil
1 cup cherry tomatoes
½ teaspoon ground black pepper
½ cup Parmesan cheese

Vegetable Soup

This recipe is super-easy, and it can be made into many other soups simply by adding more ingredients. Try adding cooked beans, barley, chicken, or beef to the sautéing onions. Or throw in a handful of pasta at the end.

1. Heat olive oil in a large sauce pan over high heat. Sauté onion, celery, carrot, parsnips, and thyme until tender.

2. Add broth and tomatoes and simmer until carrots and parsnips are tender, about 30 minutes.

3. Add peas, beans, and broccoli and simmer another 5 minutes before serving.

SERVES 4

220 calories
7 g fat
34 g carbohydrates
5 g protein
1,530 mg sodium
9 g fiber

INGREDIENTS
*2 tablespoons olive oil
1 small yellow onion, chopped
2 stalks celery, chopped
1 carrot, chopped
2 parsnips, chopped
1 teaspoon dried thyme
6 cups vegetable broth
2 cups fresh or canned
    tomatoes, chopped
1 cup fresh or frozen peas
1 cup fresh or frozen green
    beans
1 cup fresh or frozen chopped
    broccoli*

Turkey Loaf

This is an American classic, even with turkey. Some folks like to top it off with ketchup or barbecue sauce, either before or after the oven. If that's you, look for low-sodium, low-sugar sauces, or try the recipes in Chapter 5.

1. Preheat oven to 350°F.

2. Place bread in a large bowl and pour the milk on top of it. Set aside to soften for 15 minutes.

3. Stir in egg, garlic powder, onion powder, oregano, basil, and chili powder to form a paste. Add the meat and mix well.

4. Pack the meat into a loaf pan, rounding the top like a loaf of bread. Bake until brown and bubbly, about 45 minutes. If topping with sauce, add it here, and bake an additional 10 minutes to brown.

SERVES 4

350 calories
16 g fat
14 g carbohydrates
37 g protein
320 mg sodium
1 g fiber

INGREDIENTS

2 slices sandwich bread or 1 cup bread scraps or crumbs
½ cup milk
1 egg
¼ teaspoon garlic powder
¼ teaspoon onion powder
½ teaspoon dried oregano
½ teaspoon dried basil
½ teaspoon chili powder
1½ pounds ground turkey

Soft Tacos

SERVES 4–6

1,350 calories
109 g fat
53 g carbohydrates
46 g protein
810 mg sodium
12 g fiber

INGREDIENTS
1 bunch cilantro, chopped
5 cloves garlic, chopped
1 bunch green onions,
    chopped
1–3 jalapeño chilies, chopped
1 tablespoon ground cumin
1 teaspoon black pepper
2 cups olive oil
Zest and juice of 6 limes
Zest and juice of 1 orange
2–3 pounds beef skirt, flank,
    or chuck steaks
12–24 corn or whole-wheat
    tortillas
2–3 cups shredded lettuce
2–3 cups tomato salsa
1 cup light sour cream
2–3 cups guacamole

1. In a large zipper bag combine cilantro, garlic, onions, jalapeños, cumin, and pepper. Stir well.

2. Add oil, lime, and orange and stir.

3. Add steaks, massage in the marinade, close, and refrigerate 4 hours or overnight.

4. Remove steaks from the bag and discard any remaining marinade. Preheat grill or broiler on high heat. Grill steaks over direct high heat until browned, about 5–10 minutes per side. Remove from heat, cover with foil, and rest 5 minutes. Slice into thin strips against the grain.

5. Wrap tortillas in foil and warm in a 200°F oven. Serve buffet style with meat, warm tortillas, lettuce, salsa, sour cream, and guacamole.

Easy Guacamole
Guacamole is easy. Cut three avocados in half, remove the pit, and scoop out the fruit. Mash with a pinch of salt and the juice of one lime. Cover with plastic wrap pressed directly on the surface until ready to serve.

Vanilla Pound Cake with Mixed Berries

This pound cake is vanilla, but it can be jazzed up
with any number of flavors. Try adding lemon or
orange zest, raisins, nuts, or blueberries.

1. Preheat oven to 325°F. Coat a 9" × 6" loaf pan with pan spray.

2. Sift together flour, baking powder, and salt and set aside.

3. In a large bowl with a sturdy spoon or electric mixer, cream together the butter and ¾ cup honey until light and fluffy.

4. Add vanilla and eggs, one by one.

5. Add milk and slowly add the sifted ingredients, combining well.

6. Pour the batter into the loaf pan and bake for 45–60 minutes, until a toothpick inserted at the center of the cake comes out clean. Cool 10 minutes before inverting onto a rack. Cool completely before slicing.

7. Combine the berries in a small saucepan with remaining honey, and warm over medium heat until juicy and bubbly. Serve a slice of pound cake with a scoop of warm berries over the top.

A Pound of History
This cake is so-named because the original recipe called for a pound of each ingredient; eggs, sugar, flour, and butter. The batter was beaten vigorously (by hand) to incorporate air, which was the sole leavening (this was before baking soda or powder). Baking the cake in the traditional manner yields a dense, but delicious loaf. In the 1950s Sara Lee made a delicious light and buttery pound cake available to the masses.

SERVES 8

560 calories
26 g fat
76 g carbohydrates
8 g protein
180 mg sodium
5 g fiber

INGREDIENTS
2¼ cups cake flour
1 teaspoon baking powder
¼ teaspoon salt
8 ounces (2 sticks) butter
1 cup honey, divided
1 tablespoon vanilla
4 eggs
2 tablespoons fat-free milk
1 pint blackberries
1 pint raspberries
1 pint strawberries

Chapter 18

Adult Nutrition

Chances are that you know how your nutrition stacks up to the healthy guidelines outlined in Chapter 2. The fact that you are reading a nutrition book is a good indication that you may be ready for a change. Now that you've read all about children and teen nutritional needs, it's time to learn about yourself. This chapter includes all the basic guidelines, as well as information specific to men and women, for the average adult. You'll also find information about certain medical conditions and about what to eat as you get older.

Common Diet Mistakes

Most people already know that they should limit the fast food and increase the veggies. But there are other diet habits that affect overall nutrition that you may not have considered. Altering a few simple habits can drastically improve your general health.

Skipped Meals

Demands on our time, such as hectic work schedules, often make it challenging to sit and eat. But it is nearly impossible to eat all the recommended foods if you subtract an entire meal from the day. If you find yourself rushing out the door without breakfast or working through lunch or dinner, it is worth taking a few minutes in the morning, or the night before, to pack yourself some healthy foods to take on the road.

A simple PB&J, an apple, a box of raisins, carrot sticks, and nuts are all simple, easily transported foods that require no special preparation and pack a nutritional punch. Fueling yourself is a vital component of a successful day. If you are running on empty, you are not performing to your full potential. What's more, your overall nutrition is suffering because you are not getting the recommended daily amounts of nutrients.

Another problem with skipping meals is the hunger it leads to. When you finally have time to eat, it often includes binging.

Slow Down

It takes your stomach twenty minutes to relay the full feeling to your brain. People that eat an entire meal within the twenty minute time frame do not feel full, even though they have eaten enough. This causes overeating, and eventually discomfort. Overeating is the prime factor of weight gain, so by slowing down, caloric intake is reduced.

If slowing down is difficult, there are a few tricks to try:

- Never take a bite before the last one is swallowed completely.
- Put the fork down in between bites and chew thoroughly.

- Use the napkin and take a sip of water before taking another bite. Not only does this slow everything down, but it increases your fluid intake, which is good.
- It's rude to talk with your mouth full, so try to engage in some lively mealtime conversation. You'll slow down while simultaneously impressing others with your wit and wisdom.

Portion Size

One of the main reasons people eat too much is that they serve themselves too much food. It is easy to do if you begin a meal famished. Restaurants contribute to this too. They want to give people their money's worth, they want you to be satisfied, and they want you to return.

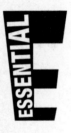

Eating the correct portion size is not difficult. There is no need to measure out your food at every meal. Simply use the palm of your hand to estimate the appropriate serving size of each food on your plate. (Read more about portion size in Chapter 2.)

Snacks

Snacking is a great way to balance out your diet. It provides an opportunity to eat extra nutrients you may be missing. It can also help curb hunger in the middle of the day and prevent binge eating at your regular meals.

Snacking should include the typical missing nutrients found in whole grains and fresh vegetables. If you are eating anything else as a snack, chances are it is doing you more harm than good. Cookies and milk, chips, pastries, blended smoothies, and coffee drinks all carry too much sugar and fat and should be limited. Instead, try air-popped popcorn, fresh vegetable sticks, a salad, dried fruits, or a bowl of cereal.

Nonfat and Sugar Free

Many people assume that nonfat or sugar-free products can be consumed in unlimited quantities. But these foods are not calorie free, and typically what they lack in one nutrient they make up for in another. For instance, sugar-free products often contain more fat and calories than their full-sugar and full-fat counterparts. And fat-free foods often compensate for lack of fat with more sugar. Read labels carefully, and remember portion control.

Instead of looking for fat-free and sugar-free versions of your favorite foods, look for nutrient-dense foods. These are foods high in vitamins, minerals, fiber, and complex carbohydrates, but low in calories. Fruits, vegetables, and whole grains fit the bill. If you are not incorporating enough of these foods in your diet, it's time to start.

Daily Eating Patterns

There is one excellent solution in the struggle to control portion size, speed eating, and junk food snacking. By eliminating the three large meals a day and replacing them with six smaller meals, you maintain a satisfied feeling and are able to fit a wider variety of foods into the daily diet. Eating a little bit every two to three hours keeps you fueled throughout the day, and makes digestion easier. This may be hard to accomplish when the rest of the family sits down to a big meal, but it may be worth some experimenting.

Alcohol

There is no good reason to include alcohol in a balanced diet. While it is true that some alcoholic beverages contain healthful ingredients, there is nothing that cannot be obtained by eating the foods recommended in this book.

The more alcohol you drink, the worse your overall nutrition is. Extra nutrients are needed to repair cells damaged by alcohol, and to strengthen normal body functions weakened by alcohol. Alcohol interferes with the body's ability to utilize the nutrients it does receive and impairs its ability to control blood glucose levels. Additionally, individuals who eat a high-fat diet accompanied by alcohol tend to overeat.

As with all foods that do not meet nutritional requirements, moderation is the key to enjoying alcohol as a part of a healthy lifestyle.

Women's Needs

Because women experience menstruation once a month, an increase in iron is necessary due to blood loss. The recommended amount of iron for middle-aged women is 18 mg per day, but many women are iron deficient. Symptoms of iron deficiency include weakness and fatigue, and deficiency can lead to anemia. Remember that vitamin C is essential for proper iron absorption. Regular periods, combined with low dietary iron and low vitamin C, commonly result in iron deficiency. After menopause, iron requirements decrease, and the recommendation drops to 10 mg.

Premenstrual syndrome (PMS) affects many women in a variety of ways. Some cases are mild, some severe. Symptoms include moodiness, bloating, tender breasts, headache, weight gain, and food cravings. A healthy diet full of complex carbohydrates and calcium can help to alleviate some of the cravings, as can regular exercise. Avoiding certain foods, including alcohol, caffeine, refined sugar, sodium, and fat, can also help.

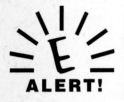

Even in the absence of hormone replacement, decreased bone density is an issue for aging women, and calcium intake should be between 1,000 and 1,500 mg a day. If you feel you cannot achieve this level of calcium through your diet, consider a calcium supplement. (Read about minerals in Chapter 5.)

Menopause, which typically begins around the age of fifty, signals the end of a woman's childbearing years. Egg production stops, and hormone production is reduced. The process can begin as early as age thirty-five, with symptoms such as insomnia, short-term memory loss, "fuzzy brain," depression, and anxiety. As the ovaries' production of progesterone and estrogen decreases, more symptoms occur, including hot flashes during the day and night, fatigue, difficulty sleeping, and mood swings.

Over the past several decades women have been given hormone replacements to ease these symptoms and increase overall health. But recently these drugs have been associated with an increase in breast cancer, heart disease, stroke, and blood clots. These findings, coupled with the side effects of hormone replacements, which include weight gain, hair loss, depression, rosacea, and a higher risk of osteoporosis, have encouraged many women to seek other forms of relief.

Natural remedies, including increased intake of vitamins E and C, have been shown to reduce the severity of hot flashes and mood swings, and magnesium seems to alleviate some women's anxiety, irritability, and panic attacks. As always, consult a physician before beginning any vitamin therapy.

Men's Needs

Most major health issues that concern men are directly associated with diet and nutrition, and are easily remedied.

Heart disease is the leading cause of death among men. This startling fact is overshadowed only by the fact that two-thirds of the male population never bothers to have their cholesterol checked. It is an easy test, and since dangerous cholesterol levels are easily remedied through diet and exercise, it's worth a simple blood test. (Read more about cholesterol in Chapter 8.)

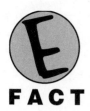

Nitrates (nitric acid salt) are used to kill microbes and preserve color in foods, especially processed meats. Your body can convert nitrates to a cancer-causing chemical called nitrosamine. Vitamin C can weaken the conversion in your stomach, but it's best to look for nitrate-free products.

Prostate cancer and colorectal cancer are two predominant male health problems, yet half of the male population is not aware of the warning signs, and many are too embarrassed to discuss the issue with their doctors.

Colon cancer is more likely to occur in men with a diet high in protein and animal fat and low in calcium. Nitrites, excessive sodium, sugar, and alcohol (more than two drinks daily) also increase risk. Obesity also puts men at risk. Early symptoms may include abdominal pain, blood in stool, or changes in bowel habits. Men over forty should begin regular screening, especially if there is a history of cancer in the family.

Prostate cancer does not typically exhibit warning signs, but a few symptoms are associated with it, including urinary frequency and urgency, slow stream, and difficulty emptying the bladder. Blood in urine is another sign, although that could indicate several problems and should be attended to immediately. Regular prostate exams should begin at age fifty, or earlier if there is a history of cancer in the family.

Herbal remedies for benign enlarged prostate include the herb saw palmetto. Zinc helps regulate testosterone in the prostate. Ginseng, also known as "man's root," is said to increase male hormone production and physical stamina. Men concerned about strength and energy can include the B-complex vitamins, which are vital to conversion of energy from foods. Be sure to discuss all supplements, herbal or otherwise, with your doctor.

Cancer Connection

Cancer is an abnormal cell that multiplies out of control, creating tumors that invade healthy tissue and spread. Carcinogens are substances that encourage development of cancer cells. They can come from the environment, food, or from within the body, and they can take years to develop.

One-third of cancer deaths are directly related to diet. Substances called inhibitors can keep these abnormal cells from growing. Many plant-based vitamins are inhibitors. Following some basic dietary guidelines, many of which are discussed at length in this book, can reduce cancer risks.

Fighting Foods

A diet containing high amounts of fiber and complex carbohydrates is a key element of reducing the risk of cancer.

Whole grains and fresh vegetables and fruits are recommended. Choices should be varied, but certain elements are beneficial in fighting particular cancers.

Fiber reduces the risk of cancers in the digestive tract, particularly colorectal cancer. Because fiber is not digested, it sweeps through the digestive tract, taking carcinogens with it. Aim for twenty to thirty grams a day of fiber. Fiber also binds with estrogen in the intestines and removes it. Without fiber, estrogen is reabsorbed and becomes a contributing factor to breast cancer.

Veggie Power

Eat plenty of bright vegetables, especially those that are orange, yellow, and red, and dark, leafy greens. Some red-pigmented fruits and vegetables, including tomatoes, pink grapefruit, watermelon, guava, and papaya, contain lycopene, a plant chemical with a strong antioxidant effect that seems to slow cancer growth, particularly when eaten fresh. Many also contain vitamin C, which is an important antioxidant that can neutralize harmful nitrates before they become carcinogenic.

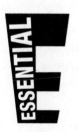

Green tea contains polyphenols, substances that interrupt the growth of cancer cells and prevent normal cells from turning cancerous. They also inhibit angiogenesis, a process by which tumor cells form blood vessels and grow. It takes a lot of tea to see these benefits, up to eight glasses a day, so many doctors suggest tea extracts.

Cabbage family (cruciferous) vegetables, including kale, broccoli, cauliflower, and brussels sprouts, contain sulforaphane, a substance that cleans up the damage done to cells by carcinogens (cancer-causing substances). It appears to be most helpful when eaten on a regular basis, as its effects are strongest when carcinogens are most active and tumors are just beginning to grow. Aim for five servings from the cabbage family every week (just cutting a little cabbage into a daily salad would do the trick).

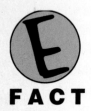

Populations that subsist on a plant-based diet, mainly underdeveloped countries where meat is scarce, have a lower rate of colon cancer. Rice and other grains are cheaper and easier to prepare and store. Throughout history mush and porridge have been the mainstay of the poor.

Good Health Sense

Obesity is a major risk factor for many cancers. To maintain a healthy weight, avoid saturated fat and foods with high cholesterol. Excessive fat is a major contributor to breast cancer, prostate cancer, colorectal cancer, as well as heart disease. Bile acid, which is secreted to digest fat, mixes with bacteria in the intestines and creates chemicals that may promote colon cancer. Dietary guidelines recommend that 30 percent of daily calories come from fat. But for those concerned with optimum health, 10–15 percent is preferred. Of that amount, the majority should be mono and polyunsaturated fats.

Avoid excess sugar and sodium. Snack foods high in sugar contain empty calories and leave less room for nutrient-rich foods. Sodium is a contributor to hypertension. Excessive alcohol consumption contributes to mouth, throat, esophagus, and liver cancers. Smoking increases these risks and causes its own problems, including lung cancer.

Other precautions include avoiding unnecessary X-rays, staying out of direct sunlight, taking estrogen only when absolutely necessary, and adhering to health and safety regulations in the workplace. And as always, exercise regularly.

Diabetes

Diabetes mellitus is a disorder of the metabolism resulting in abnormal blood sugar levels, called hyperglycemia. It is caused by low levels of insulin or a resistance to the effects of insulin.

Type I diabetes, also known as insulin dependent, or juvenile onset, diabetes is caused by the inability of the pancreas to produce sufficient insulin. Although the cause is unknown, it is believed to be an autoimmune reaction to a virus or bacterial infection.

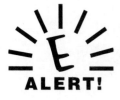

Food-borne chemical toxins and exposure to cow's milk at too early an age are thought to trigger the autoimmune reactions related to type I diabetes. This is why cow's milk appears on the list of foods to avoid in the first year of life.

Type II diabetes, also known as noninsulin dependent, or adult onset, diabetes, occurs when insulin cannot trigger the conversion of food to energy. This is the most common form of diabetes. Age, obesity, and physical inactivity are major causes. It can also be caused by illness that damages the pancreas. Gestational diabetes occurs in pregnant women, but usually disappears after the birth of the baby.

Prediabetes conditions include a higher than normal blood sugar level, which can be treated through diet and exercise. More serious diabetes symptoms include excessive thirst; irregular urination; weight loss; blurred vision; excessive hunger; skin, bladder, and gum infections; numbness in feet; slow-healing wounds; and extreme fatigue. Risk is highest in overweight, inactive people over forty-five, or those with a family history of the disease.

Diabetes patients are the most likely to develop heart disease and stroke. Diabetes is the leading cause of blindness, kidney disease, limb amputation, and nerve damage. It is the sixth leading cause of death in the United States.

The best weapon against diabetes is a healthy diet and plenty of regular exercise. Follow the dietary guidelines recommended in Chapter 2, which include getting plenty of whole grains, fresh vegetables, fruits, and low-fat dairy and protein and keeping sugar to a moderate amount.

Hypertension

High blood pressure, or hypertension, is often referred to as the silent killer because there are no symptoms and it can go undetected until it is too late. Blood pressure is the force put on the artery walls by flowing blood. Blood pressure is measured in millimeters of mercury (mmHg), which indicates how high the pressure of the blood will raise a column of mercury. There are two measurements; the systolic, which measures the pressure at each pulse beat, and the diastolic, which measures the pressure between each beat.

Reading Blood Pressure

	systolic	diastolic
Normal	< 120 mmHg	< 80 mmHg
Warning	120–139 mmHg	80–89 mmHg
Phase 1 Hypertension	140–159 mmHg	90–99 mmHg
Phase 2 Hypertension	> 160 mmHg	> 100

Blood pressure is read as systolic/diastolic. For example, normal blood pressure would be read 120/80.

Potassium works with sodium to regulate the body's water balance. (Read more about electrolytes in Chapter 5.) Diets low in calcium are also at a higher risk for hypertension. By decreasing sodium (no more than 1,500–2,300 mg per day), increasing natural forms of potassium, and maintaining a normal weight through a healthy diet, hypertension may be decreased.

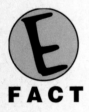

FACT

Reminder: One teaspoon of table salt contains 2,000 milligrams of sodium. Most Americans consume 4,000–6,000 milligrams of salt every day. The recommended daily limit of salt is 2,400 milligrams, but your body only needs about 400 milligrams (less than a quarter teaspoon).

The DASH diet

The Dietary Approach to Stopping Hypertension (DASH) is a diet high in potassium, calcium, and magnesium. It encourages foods that are high in fiber and complex carbohydrates and low in fat. Studies have shown the DASH diet to significantly reduce blood pressure after eight weeks.

DASH Diet Daily Recommended Servings:

- 7–8 servings whole grains
- 4–5 servings vegetables
- 4–5 servings fruits
- 2–3 servings low-fat dairy
- < 2 servings lean meat
- 4–5 servings nuts, seeds, and legumes

Heart Disease

There are a number of abnormal heart conditions affecting the heart and blood vessels that are characterized as heart disease. Most can be avoided with a healthy diet and exercise.

Coronary Artery Disease

Coronary artery disease is the most common cause of heart attacks. It is characterized by the buildup of LDL cholesterol (known as arterial plaque), which hardens and narrows arteries, and slows down blood flow. (Read more about arterial blockage in Chapter 8.)

Angina

Arterial blockage from plaque can lead to angina, which is a squeezing pain in the chest, jaw, arms, shoulder, neck, and back. Angina is a warning sign of a potential heart attack.

Heart Attack

Actual heart attacks occur when the artery is blocked and the heart cannot get the blood it needs for over twenty minutes.

Heart Failure

Heart failure is the inability of the heart to pump blood adequately. It is not a case of the heart stopping, but rather of other organs not getting the blood they need. Symptoms include shortness of breath; swelling in the legs, ankles, and feet; and extreme fatigue.

Heart Arrhythmia

Arrhythmia is characterized by a change in the beats of the heart, which can cause dizziness, chest pain, and shortness of breath. The changing pattern and accompanying symptoms usually occur separately and are harmless. But if they occur simultaneously they can be very dangerous.

To reduce the risk of heart disease, know your blood pressure, and if necessary, take steps to lower it by instituting the DASH diet. Eat a healthy diet, exercise regularly, and maintain a healthy weight. Check cholesterol regularly, don't smoke, and limit alcohol to one drink a day. Overweight individuals are at a higher risk for heart disease, as are those with diabetes.

Gastrointestinal Disorders

A diet high in fiber and water can help prevent several diseases that attack the gastrointestinal system.

Diverticulitis

This disease is characterized by pouches that form in the wall of the colon from pressure exerted on weak spots. Symptoms include abdominal pain, cramping, and diarrhea. A diet low in fiber forces the colon to work harder, exerting more pressure on the walls as stool is moved through. Stool remaining in the bowel longer also exerts more pressure. A high-fiber diet is often recommended for people with this condition.

Gallstones

As tiny as a grain of sand, or as big as a walnut, gallstones are bits of cholesterol in the bile. Symptoms depend on the number and size of gallstones. If they move into and block ducts that connect the gallbladder, pancreas, and liver with the intestines, they create pain, infection, and organ damage. Symptoms include pain in the upper right belly, which can spread to the back and shoulder. It may or may not be severe, and it may feel worse after meals. Keeping at a healthy weight by eating a balanced diet high in fiber and calcium, with limited saturated fat and cholesterol, can reduce risk of gallstones.

Ulcers

Ulcers are sores on the inner lining of the stomach and upper small intestine (the duodenum). The protective layer of the stomach is broken down and irritated by gastric juices, which include hydrochloric acid and the enzyme pepsin. Symptoms, which can come and go, include abdominal pain, burning and aching of the belly, back pain, bloating, and nausea after meals. Alcohol slows the healing of ulcers and increases symptoms. Remedies include ending tobacco, caffeine, and alcohol consumption and reducing stress.

Eating As You Age

All body systems decline as you age, and all of these changes can adversely affect overall nutrition. You lose lean muscle mass, which includes the mass of your cardiac muscle. Your metabolic rate declines, you have reduced body water, and your body fat increases, especially around the trunk, where the vital organs are. Osteoporosis can become severely debilitating as bone density decreases, especially in postmenopausal women.

Because people become less active and their muscles aren't worked very hard, calorie intake needs to be adjusted. The trick is to get the same amount of nutrients in fewer calories. This makes getting a proper diet difficult for the elderly. Diminished senses can make matters worse.

Eyesight deteriorates, and loss of clear vision can make the elderly timid around the stove. They are less likely to read menus, recipes, and labels clearly. Hearing loss often results in a reluctance to ask questions of waiters or grocers, which in turn results in less shopping and dining out. Diminished sense of taste makes food less appetizing, and dietary restrictions on sodium and sugar don't help.

Many elderly find themselves eating alone and tend to skip meals as appetites decrease and preparation becomes more difficult. Poorly fitted dentures frequently cause pain, which makes eating unpleasant. Coupled with bland, mushy preparation, malnutrition can become a serious problem among the aged.

This is a time of life when good nutrition can drastically improve the quality of life. Seeking out quality meals should be a priority. Take advantage of frozen or premade meals with easy preparations. Seek out local organizations that deliver meals. To combat the bland diet, experiment with new food, textures, and flavors by sampling international and exotic cuisines. Try some of the many salt substitutes to add flavor back into your food. (Try some of the recipes in Chapter 5.)

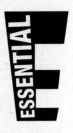

In addition to extra calcium, regular exercise is vital to maintaining bone strength. Walk, swim, or lift weights at least three times a week. Look for fitness classes geared toward seniors at the local YMCA, senior center, or recreation department.

Choose foods high in nutrients but low in calories. Sixty percent of calories should come from complex carbohydrates. Be sure to get adequate fiber and water, and choose low-fat dairy and protein sources. Increase calcium by eating two to four servings of nonfat or low-fat dairy foods every day. Women may need a calcium supplement. Milk enriched with vitamin D is especially important for housebound seniors, or those that do not venture into the sunshine often. Zinc is an important nutrient for slowing muscular degeneration, and vitamin C is important for calcium and iron absorption. Lack of vitamin B_{12} and folic acid are associated with hearing loss, and vitamin E is thought to reduce the risk of Alzheimer's disease.

Chapter 19

Special Diets

More and more people are watching what they eat, and that's a good thing. But there are a lot of crazy fads out there, as well as thousands of products designed to make you healthy and fit. Sifting through all of that may seem daunting, but armed with basic nutritional information, it can all make sense.

Dieting Versus Your Diet

A diet is the food you eat. Dieting is a specific selection of food chosen to aid in weight loss, weight gain, or meeting particular nutritional needs. Your diet is initially determined by your culture, but dietary habits can easily be altered to address health and moral issues.

There are several reasons people elect to change their dietary habits. The most common is weight loss, as is evidenced by the multibillion-dollar weight-loss industry. Health is another factor, as people discover that eating habits are responsible for, and can help correct, illness and disease. People also choose special diets for peace of mind, whether they are morally against eating animals or religiously bound to culinary tradition and rules.

Fasting is a bad idea. Starving yourself may drop a few pounds initially, but you are only losing water and muscle mass. You will most likely gain it right back, and the lack of nourishment can cause physical damage, including gallstones (see Chapter 18).

High-Protein, Low-Carb

The principle subscribed to by this plan is that overeating is directly caused by carbohydrates, which do not initially satisfy and thus create further cravings. When carbohydrates are restricted, people spontaneously reduce the number of calories they eat, simply because they are not hungry. Intake eventually corresponds to natural levels appropriate for the person's height.

Atkins Diet

This diet, designed by Dr. Robert Atkins in the 1960s, was built on the idea that obesity is a direct result of refined carbohydrates such as sugar, white flour, and high-fructose corn syrup. He also believed that saturated fat is not nearly as bad as trans fat from partially hydrogenated vegetable oil. The theory of the diet is that by restricting carbohydrates, the body's metabolism switches from burning glucose for fuel to burning body fat.

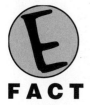

FACT

When the body burns fat instead of glucose, it is called lipolysis. Burning fat for energy creates by-products called ketone bodies, which can be used as a source of energy in the heart and brain. When carbohydrates are sufficiently restricted, the body moves into what is known as a state of ketosis, and weight loss occurs.

The Atkins diet involves limiting "net carbs," which are counted by subtracting sugar alcohols and fiber from the total carbohydrates. Fructose is also limited. Protein and fat is unlimited, and the twenty to twenty-five grams of carbohydrates allowed per day are taken in the form of green vegetables.

Since its introduction, the Atkins diet has been criticized as unhealthy, although there are no studies to support this criticism.

The Zone

This diet is often lumped into the low-carb bracket, but its creator, Barry Sears, insists it is not low carbohydrates but proper hormone balance that is the key to the Zone diet.

The Zone refers to the proper ratio of carbohydrates, protein, and fat, 40:30:30, which emphasizes a decrease in unhealthy carbohydrates (rather than an increase in protein). Carbohydrates considered unhealthy are the same as those frowned on by the Atkins plan: refined sugar, white flour, and high-fructose corn syrup.

The Zone includes fat based on the belief that fat must be consumed in order to burn fat. The theory is that low-fat diets increase insulin production, which causes the body to store fat. Fat in the Zone diet is mainly unsaturated.

South Beach

This diet, created by Miami cardiologist Arthur Agatston, emphasizes "good carbs" and "good fats." Carbohydrates with a high glycemic index are thought to create "insulin resistance syndrome," in which insulin is unable to properly process fats and sugars. By eliminating easily absorbed sugars, as well as saturated fats and trans fats, the risk of heart disease is reduced, and weight loss results.

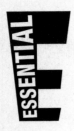

The glycemic index rates carbohydrates based on their effect on blood sugar levels. Fruit has a low glycemic index number of 55 or below. Candy is considered medium, with a glycemic index of between 55 and 69. Starches have the highest glycemic index at 70 or above. The higher the number, the faster blood glucose levels will rise, which translates to fast, short bursts of energy.

Paleolithic Diet

This diet revolves around the notion that human genetics have changed little since the Stone Age and that the best foods for you are those you were designed to eat. Anything that can be hunted or gathered, and prepared with minimal cooking, is the mainstay of this diet. It works in a similar manner to the Atkins diet, focusing on meat, fish, eggs, vegetables, fruits, nuts, and seeds.

Allergies and Intolerances

Food sensitivities are classified as either an allergy or intolerance. Both mean that certain foods must be eliminated from the diet, but the reactions occur in different body functions.

Food allergies are an immune system response. The food is interpreted by the body as an attacking substance, usually remembered from a previous exposure, and the body reacts by sending antibodies to fight it. The resulting symptoms can be mild, or life threatening, and include rash, hives, chest pain, shortness of breath, swelling of airways, and anaphylaxis.

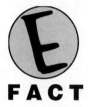

FACT

Anaphylaxis is an allergic reaction that occurs from eating, breathing, touching, or injecting an allergen. The name comes from the Greek *ana,* meaning "against," and *phylaxis,* meaning "protection." Symptoms can be mild or severe, ranging from swelling, itching, vomiting, fainting, and difficulty breathing to a sudden drop in blood pressure. Severe symptoms can result in death within minutes if not treated immediately.

Food intolerance is a response from the digestive system and is usually not life threatening. Intolerance occurs if the body does not possess the enzymes or chemicals it needs to break down a food and digest it. Symptoms are unpleasant and can cause illness and long-term health problems.

With both allergies and intolerances, the severity of the reaction varies with the individual.

The most common food sensitivities have prompted the creation of a variety of products to support a normal and varied diet. Manufacturers are continually creating new foods made without the most common problematic ingredients. Cross-contamination is a particular issue, and more and more products are being manufactured separately to prevent accidental exposure.

People who suffer from these problems must learn to read labels carefully and get in the habit of asking friends what is in the food they are cooking. Dining at restaurants is considerably more difficult. Calling ahead to discuss allergies is a typical approach, and these sensitive diners tend to stick with the restaurants they find accommodating.

Dairy

Dairy products cause both allergies and intolerances. Milk allergy is an immune system response to milk protein. This is the most common allergy found in infants and young children, but they often outgrow it. Symptoms include rashes, hives, gastrointestinal distress, and breathing problems. Anaphylaxis is rare. Those suffering from milk allergies must avoid all dairy products, foods made with dairy products, and foods containing whey or casein.

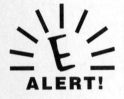

Casein is a protein in milk that is used in food manufacturing as a binder. It can appear in nondairy foods, such as soy cheese or nondairy creamer, so milk-sensitive people need to look for casein on food labels.

Intolerance to dairy is specifically an intolerance to milk sugar, or lactose. The body is missing lactase, an enzyme needed to digest milk sugar. Several hours after eating dairy, bloating, abdominal pain, gas, and diarrhea occur. Some who are lactose intolerant can consume foods with trace amounts of dairy. Yogurt does not cause distress because its amazing bacteria helps to consume lactose fast—so fast that the body doesn't have time to react to having eaten it.

There are several dairy products on the market that are specially treated for the lactose intolerant, such as lactose-free cheese, milk, and ice cream. For allergies, all milk products must be avoided. Substitutes include soy, rice, and almond milks, margarine, and a host of other nondairy products, including ice cream, chocolate, cheese, and yogurt. Calcium is an essential element of the diet that must be replaced with calcium-rich vegetables and supplements.

Wheat and Gluten

There are several proteins in wheat that can cause an allergy or intolerance. These proteins give wheat its unique elasticity and make it an excellent binder. For that reason, wheat flour is found in a surprising amount of foods, including ketchup and ice cream. Those with sensitivities must become expert label readers.

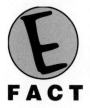

FACT

Gluten is the most common cause of wheat sensitivity. Gluten is composed of two proteins, glutenin and gliadin. Together, when moistened and agitated, they create elasticity. This elasticity, among other things, allows bread dough to rise.

An allergy or intolerance to a specific protein may include other grains in the same family as wheat (triticea), including barley, rye, and oats. Wheat is also found in other forms that go by different names, including farina, bran, graham, bulgur, durum, semolina, malt, and starch.

To cook without wheat, substitute one tablespoon of wheat flour with one and a half teaspoons (i.e., half the amount) of cornstarch, potato starch, arrowroot starch, rice flour, or tapioca. Larger quantities of flour can be replaced with a more or less equal amount of corn meal, potato flour, or rice flour. Substitution ratios will vary depending on the recipe, so experimentation is recommended.

Celiac disease is an autoimmune disorder of the small bowel. Two wheat proteins, gliadin and glutenin, cannot be modified by enzymes, and the immune system reacts with inflammation that interferes with the absorption of nutrients. Luckily, there are many gluten-free food options available today.

Nuts

Peanuts and tree nuts are among the most common food allergies. They are so common that nut-free products, restaurants, and even schools are becoming commonplace.

Nut allergies can be severe. Symptoms can include tingling mouth and lips, hives, swelling in the throat, asthma, vomiting, cramps, anaphylaxis, fainting, and unconsciousness. Death can occur as a result of obstruction of airways and extremely low blood pressure.

Like wheat, nuts are found in an enormous number of products. As of 2006, labels are required to clearly state if a product contains nuts. Watch for nut-derived ingredients in soup, gravy, chili, ice cream, chocolate, and candy, as well as pet foods and bedding.

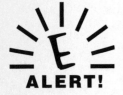

ALERT!

It is possible to be cross-contaminated by your pets. Pet bedding and food commonly contain nut derivatives. If you have a severe allergy to nuts, look for nut-free dog food, or you may find yourself faced with potentially hazardous drool.

Nut oils are difficult to remove by washing, so cross-contamination of nut residue is a real concern. Avoid buffet dining, in which ladles and serving utensils can migrate between foods. Avoid dining out on cuisines that are known to use lots of nuts, including Asian, African, and Mexican. Avoid fried foods, as fryer oil often contains peanut oil. Above all, teach your friends and family to recognize anaphylaxis.

Religious Restrictions

Many religions include dietary laws. Jewish and Muslim dietary laws are similar, one following the Law of Moses, the other keeping in step with the notion of clean and unclean. Hindus are mainly vegetarian, as are Buddhists, although meat and fish are allowed following strict guidelines. Early Christian food rules banned the consumption of meat offered to idols, blood, and things that were strangled. Roman Catholics abstained from meat on Fridays until the Second Vatican Council (Vatican II) in the 1960s.

Kosher Foods

Kosher is the English word for *kashrut*, or the Hebrew dietary laws derived from the Torah's book of Leviticus. Foods that are not kosher are *treif*. The only animals that may be eaten are those deemed clean, which include quadrupeds that chew their cud and have completely split hoofs, fish with both fins and scales, domesticated birds, locusts, and grasshoppers.

Kosher slaughter and preparation of food is strictly regulated. Animals must be killed in a clean and humane manner to limit the animal's suffering and demonstrate the responsibility that comes with having power over life and death. In preparing meat, body fat and sinuous tendons must be removed, and the body must be drained completely of all fluids.

Specific food combinations are prohibited. An animal may not be seethed (boiled) in its mother's milk. This act is seen as a symbolic combination of life and death and is interpreted in modern times as the prohibition of meat and milk in any form being cooked or eaten together. This includes food in the same dish or within the same meal. Fish and meat are also not to be consumed together, and there are certain holidays that require specific foods.

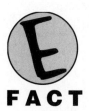

FACT

Following kosher law is an act of faith, although many scholars continue to explore the health benefits of the kosher diet. It appears to be a more hygienic, less toxic diet overall.

Kosher foods in the market are marked with a symbol that indicates they have been certified by a rabbi or rabbinical authority. Symbols include a *U*, *OU*, and *K*. In addition, foods containing specific ingredients are clearly labeled, including *D* for dairy, *P* for fish, *M* for meat, and *Pareve*, which means no meat or dairy.

Vegetarianism

Whether through love of animals or basic knowledge of nutrition, many cultures eliminate meat from their diets. Vegetarianism was recorded in ancient India and Greece as a philosophy of nonviolence, and became widely popular in Europe and the United States in the nineteenth and twentieth centuries.

There are several levels of vegetarianism. Ovo-vegetarians permit the consumption of eggs. Lacto-vegetarians permit dairy products. Some vegetarians will allow only certain animals into their diets, such as pescetarians, who will eat fish, and pollotarians, who will eat poultry. These exceptions usually stem from dietary concerns. Macrobiotic vegetarians avoid processed foods, consuming mainly whole grains and beans and occasionally seafood.

Diets that are plant-based have many benefits, especially a reduction in saturated fats and cholesterol. Additionally, these diets are high in healthful fiber, complex carbohydrates, and naturally occurring vitamins and minerals. Vegetarians report less heart disease, hypertension, and cancer. They have lower cholesterol and blood pressure and lower occurrence of dementia, including Alzheimer's disease.

The downside is the lack of protein and the care with which vegetarians must combine foods to create complete proteins. But vegetarianism is common, and there are ample products on the market that serve as meat replacements. There are also many resources to assist vegetarians in proper diet. (Read more about complete protein in Chapter 6.)

Vegan

Those who abstain from all animal products are known as vegans. This frequently includes avoiding household items and clothing made from animals in addition to animal-based food. The focus of most veganism is the ethical treatment of animals and a concern for the environment. There are a few offshoots of veganism. Raw vegans believe that cooking foods removes beneficial nutrients, and their diet excludes food cooked above 115°F. A fruitarian diet consists mainly of plants that are not damaged by harvest. The motivation for this diet is usually spiritual, including a reluctance to kill in any manner. Some fruitarians are trying to recreate a diet similar to that of Adam and Eve, with the belief that it is what God intended.

The Vegetarian Menu

Plants can supply you with all the basic nutrients if eaten in the proper combinations. A few simple guidelines will help keep the diet healthy and beneficial.

- Eat a variety of whole grains and legumes. Together, these foods create the complete protein that would otherwise be derived from meat. These foods do not have to be eaten in the same meal, but should each be consumed each day.
- Eating the same foods every day limits the vitamins and minerals you are getting. Eat a variety of fresh fruits and vegetables prepared in a manner that best utilizes their nutrients. Eating brightly colored vegetables maximizes your nutrient intake.
- Incorporate seeds and nuts into recipes. Sprinkled on salads, in cereal, and baked goods, nuts and seeds give added protein, calcium, and omega-3 oils.
- Avoid foods and preparations with excessive fats and sugars. Choose lower-fat dairy products. Limit foods with high saturated fat.
- Consider dietary supplements of nutrients found mainly in meat products, including iron, calcium, and B_{12}. Vitamin D is also a concern if dairy is eliminated.
- Use soy liberally, in the form of milk or tofu. It adds a creamy texture to foods, and boosts protein.
- Don't restrict fats in vegan and vegetarian children under the age of two. They need it for healthy growth.

The following guidelines give daily dietary needs for both vegetarians and vegans.

- **Legumes:** Two or more servings per day. These include beans, peas, lentils, tofu, and meat substitutes. Eggs can be included here for ovo-vegetarians.
- **Vegetables:** Three or more servings per day. Include dark green, leafy vegetables, such as spinach; bright orange vegetables, such as sweet potatoes; and bright red and purple vegetables, including tomatoes, beets, and purple cabbage.
- **Fruits:** Thee or more servings per day. Include citrus, melons, apples, berries, and tropical fruits. Eat the skins when possible.
- **Whole grains:** Six to eleven servings per day. Include cereals and breads, rice, and specialty grains like quinoa.

- **Dairy or fortified dairy substitutes:** Two to three servings per day. Choose low-fat dairy products, or dairy substitutes. Look for products enriched with calcium and vitamin D.
- **Fats, oils, nuts, sugar:** Use sparingly. Avoid saturated and trans fat, and choose unsaturated or polyunsaturated fats instead.
- **Supplements:** Calcium, iron, B_{12}, and omega-3 fatty acids can be obtained naturally, but consider supplements if the diet is not sufficiently varied.

Chapter 20

The Importance of Exercise

No book on nutrition would be complete without a section on exercise. That is because it is impossible to live a nutritious and healthy lifestyle without it. Humans are creatures designed to move, yet we spend the majority of the day sitting in chairs. What is this electronic revolution doing to your health?

Your Exercise Requirement

The American Heart Association recommends thirty minutes of aerobic physical activity a day at moderate intensity. Unfortunately, this guideline is misleading.

In 1995 the Centers for Disease Control and Prevention (CDC) and the American College of Sports Medicine (ACSM) made a public health recommendation that every U.S. adult should accumulate thirty minutes or more of moderate-intensity physical activity on most, preferably all, days of the week.

The recommendation seemed clear enough, but was misinterpreted by many. Some believed that higher-intensity activity would not be beneficial, while others considered it to mean that any movement would suffice. Therefore, in 2007 the following new guidelines were issued:

Healthy adults age eighteen to sixty-five need moderate-intensity aerobic physical activity of at least thirty minutes per session on five or more days per week, or vigorous-intensity aerobic activity for at least twenty minutes three or more days per week. Combinations of moderate- and vigorous-intensity activity can be performed to satisfy these requirements. In addition, every adult should perform activities that maintain or increase muscular strength and endurance a minimum of two days each week.

In order to understand these guidelines fully, it is important to understand what constitutes moderate and vigorous intensity.

Target Heart Rate

The difficulty in determining the intensity of exercise lies in the fact that everyone is different. What makes one person huff and puff will barely break a sweat on someone else. To adequately measure intensity, the target heart rate is used.

Measuring target heart rate first requires knowing your average maximum heart rate, which is determined by subtracting your age from 220. Your target heart rate is 50–85 percent of your maximum. It is a wide range. When you begin an exercise program, your target is the lower end of the range, and as you become more physically fit, you aim higher.

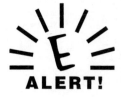

Some high-blood-pressure medications can lower your maximum heart rate. Check with your doctor to determine if your medication does this, and to find your new target heart rate.

Begin by measuring your pulse. To do this, put two fingers, preferably your second and third fingers, on your carotid or radial artery. The carotid artery is alongside your wind pipe, and your radial artery can be found in the groove of your inner wrist, below your thumb. Move your fingers around until you feel the pulse. Using a timepiece with a second hand or a stop watch, count the pulse beats for ten seconds. Multiply by six for your beats per minute (bpm). (Alternatively, you can count for six seconds and multiply by ten.)

Target Heart Rate

Age	Target Heart Rate (50–85%)	Average Maximum Heart Rate (100%)
20	100–179 bpm	200 bpm
30	89–162 bpm	190 bpm
40	90–153 bpm	180 bpm
50	85–145 bpm	170 bpm
60	80–136 bpm	160 bpm
70	75–128 bpm	150 bpm

It is possible to estimate intensity without the heart rate. It's called the chat test, and it is useful if your activity doesn't allow you to take your pulse. If you can chat easily during your activity, your intensity is low. If you can speak, but are breathing heavily, your intensity is moderate. If you can't talk at all, your intensity is high.

Body Mass Index

The body mass index (BMI) is a measurement used to determine relative body fat. The number will indicate if a person is normal weight, underweight, overweight, or obese. The BMI measurement uses weight and height in its calculation and is therefore not a method that directly measures fat. Other methods, including underwater weighing and skin fold thickness measurements, are more accurate but are also more costly. BMI provides a reliable approximation and will indicate if an individual has serious body fat issues. Then, the lifestyle can be adjusted accordingly.

To measure your BMI, multiply your weight (in pounds) by 703, then divide by your height (in inches) twice:

$$weight\ (lbs.) \times 703\ /\ height\ (inches)\ /\ height\ (inches)$$

Body Mass Index

BMI	Weight Status
< 18.5	underweight
18.5–24.9	normal weight
25.0–29.9	overweight
> 30.0	obese

Keep in mind that BMI is affected by several variables, including age, sex, race, and musculature. Older adults and women tend to have more body fat, while athletes tend to have heavy muscles. For that reason, a twenty-year-old male athlete may have the same BMI as a forty-year-old female office worker, but they may be miles apart in terms of actual fitness. The measurement is meant only as a general indication.

Calories and Basal Metabolic Rate (BMR)

Calories measure energy. They are determined by burning a measured portion of food and measuring the amount of heat (or calories) it produces. The number of calories you need depends on your Basal Metabolic Rate (BMR), your level of physical activity, and the energy you need to digest, absorb, and metabolize food.

Your BMR is the energy your body needs while awake and at rest. It varies with each individual, but can be generally determined by the following formulas:

- Male BMR = 66 + (6.21 × your weight in pounds) + (12.7 × your height in inches) − (6.8 × your age)
- Female BMR = 655 + (4.37 × your weight in pounds) + (2.32 × your height in inches) − (4.7 × your age)

To determine your daily caloric needs, multiply your BMR by the number that best represents your activity level:

Activity Level

Activity Level	BMR Multiplier
Sedentary (little or no exercise)	1.2
Lightly active (light exercise 1–3 days per week)	1.375
Moderately active (moderate activity 3–5 days per week)	1.55
Very active (heavy exercise 6–7 days per week)	1.725
Extra active (professional athlete)	1.9

Weighing Your Risk

Most people already know if they are at their ideal weight. You can see it in the mirror. But you can have a more accurate indication of how your current weight stacks up to your ideal weight.

First, determine your body frame size. Medium frame males have a seven-inch wrist. Medium frame women have a six-inch wrist. Larger frames have larger wrists, and smaller frames have smaller wrists. Now add up the pounds to determine your ideal weight:

- Medium Frame Males
  100 pounds for the first five feet of height
  5 pounds for every inch over five feet
  take away 5 pounds for every inch under five feet

- Medium Frame Females
  106 pounds for the first five feet of height
  6 pounds for every inch over five feet
  take away 6 pounds for every inch under five feet
- Smaller frames subtract 10 percent
- Larger frames add 10 percent

Weigh the Results

Now that you have a general idea of where you stand, you can begin to adjust your diet accordingly.

To lose weight, your calorie intake must be less than your current daily caloric needs. To gain weight, it must be more.

To lose weight (which is the more common goal), you need to burn about 3,500 calories more than you consume. This can be accomplished by eliminating these calories from your diet, burning more calories through exercise, or both. For example, walking fast (so you're breathing heavily) for fifteen to twenty miles a week will burn about 2,500 calories. As your fitness improves, you must increase the intensity or duration of your exercise to maintain the weight loss.

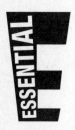

Keep challenging yourself. Taking the same walk day after day will only help you for so long. As your body becomes accustomed to the motion, and your muscles develop, the movement is no longer challenging, and your heart is no longer working hard. Pick up the pace, take a hill, or start running.

Water and Exercise

Unless you're an elite athlete, water is the best way to replenish fluids lost in exercise. Sports drinks are made to replenish lost electrolytes and provide added carbohydrates to fuel athletes after prolonged vigorous exercise. Everyday moderate exercise of thirty to forty minutes does not qualify.

Thirty minutes before you go out for your daily routine, drink one to two cups of water. Throughout your exercise, drink a half to one cup of water every ten to fifteen minutes. When you're done, replenish your fluids by slowly drinking water over the next several hours. To adequately rehydrate, you should consume two cups of water for every pound lost during exercise.

Dehydration

Water is the most abundant, and the most important, nutrient in your body. You need it to carry the other nutrients to organs, and oxygen to your cells. Blood is made mostly of water, as are your lungs, muscles, and brain. You need water to regulate your body's temperature, remove waste, and cushion your joints and organs. A lack of water can cause mental and physical problems. If water is not replenished as it is lost, you begin to see symptoms of dehydration. Regardless of how much water you drink, you are constantly losing water throughout the day in urine, perspiration, and respiration.

Perspiration is the body's natural cooling system. Sweat on the skin cools our overall body temperature as it evaporates. Respiration releases moisture with every breath you exhale. Exercising increases this type of water loss, as breathing becomes heavier and more frequent. In general, active people need more water than sedentary folks.

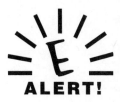

Fatigue, irritability, and headaches are some of the first noticeable symptoms of dehydration. Thirst is a later symptom, usually indicating that dehydration is well underway. Symptoms of prolonged dehydration include pain in joints, muscles, and the lower back, as well as constipation and dark urine.

Diuretics are substances that trick the body into thinking it has more water than it really does. They do this by making the kidneys generate urine. Caffeine is the most common diuretic. It causes you to lose more water than you should, causing dehydration. This is why quenching your thirst with caffeinated drinks is counterproductive.

Sugary drinks also cause dehydration. When glucose enters the blood stream it attracts water, and your body tries to compensate for the loss by making you thirsty. You can really notice this effect after eating particularly sweet foods, like ice cream.

To keep your body healthy and hydrated, water is by far the best thing to drink.

How Much Is Enough?

For years you have been told to drink eight glasses of water a day. It is a good general rule, although there has been little scientific study to support this recommendation. With water, as with other elements of good nutrition, the right amount varies with the individual.

One popular formula is to divide your body weight in two. That number is the number of ounces you should be drinking daily. If you are active, you need to add more water. If you live in a dry climate, you need to add more. If you drink alcohol you should add that amount of extra water as well.

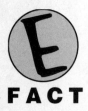

FACT

In-flight air is said to be drier than the Arabian Desert. Fifty percent humidity is a comfortable environment, but the dry airplane cabin air is typically about 1 percent. If you are traveling in an airplane, you should drink eight ounces of water every hour to combat airplane-induced dehydration. And avoid the free salty snacks. They only make matters worse.

Getting Your Family to Drink

Once you are convinced of water's importance, it's time to spread the word. This is sometimes easier said than done.

Some people find water boring and if given a choice, will choose a more interesting beverage. But the effect of water, or the lack thereof, can be seen every day. School kids are especially susceptible. They get tired and cranky when they are dehydrated. After recess, if they have not fully rehydrated, their attention drifts, and they suffer fatigue. It is not the best way to impress the teacher. When added to stress, lack of sleep, and poor nutrition, dehydration can lead to dangerous consequences behind the wheel. Avoid high-sugar and high-sodium snacks on long car trips, and always carry water, even on short trips to the market.

Teach kids to stop each time they pass a drinking fountain and take a sip. Give them refillable water bottles to drink from throughout the day.

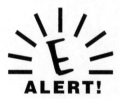

Some of the most popular, top-selling, reusable bottles in sporting good stores are made from #7 plastic. If you have these at home, wash them carefully in cool soapy water. If they have been through the dishwasher, discard them.

Adults also suffer from dehydration, especially fatigue and headaches. These symptoms can make everyday activities excruciating. If you develop the habit of sipping water throughout the day, you will notice a marked improvement in your attention and energy levels. Adequate water also improves skin, flushes toxins, and boosts the metabolism. When you're hungry, drinking a glass of water before sitting down to a meal will slow your eating and make you full faster. If you are on a low-carb, high-protein diet, extra water can help remove waste from the digestive system and help to break down stored fat. Don't forget that you get a lot of water from the food you eat. The more fresh fruits and vegetables you eat raw, before heat from cooking has had a chance to evaporate their waters, the more water you're getting.

Drinking Green

There are a number of environmental concerns about plastic bottles that hold water. Because plastic bottles are harmful to the environment, refillable bottles are the way to go. But they may not all be safe.

The controversy surrounding plastic bottles revolves around the chemical bisphenol A (BPA), a known hormone disruptor that mimics and disrupts natural hormones, including estrogen, that control brain and reproductive functions. The chemical can leach from plastic containers into food and drink. The effect is heightened with prolonged storage, and when heated (as in the dishwasher).

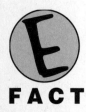

FACT

The Environmental Protection Agency (EPA) studied BPA in the 1980s, and concluded that it is only harmful when consumed in immense quantities. However, a 2006 study indicated a possible correlation between this chemical and enhanced risk of type II diabetes, ovarian dysfunction, mammary gland development, and miscarriage. The data is inconsistent, so until further studies are completed, these products are still on the market.

Plastics are labeled with a number that is an indication of the resin used in its manufacture. The initial purpose was to help identify which plastics could be recycled together. Today it also helps consumers identify safe plastics. The following table gives the plastic numbers, their makeup, and their effects.

Plastic Safety

Number	Plastic	Effect
#1	polyethylene terephthalate (PET)	human carcinogen seen only after nine months storage
#2	high-density polyethylene (HDPE)	chemical leaching probability increases with age and heat
#3	polyvinyl chloride (V or PVC)	known to release carcinogenic toxins into environment

Number	Plastic	Effect
#4	low-density polyethylene (LDPE)	low level leaching only after prolonged storage
#5	polypropylene (PP)	not known to leach dioxins or carcinogens
#6	polystyrene (PS)	leaches styrene, a possible human carcinogen and hormone disruptor
#7	polycarbonate	leaches BPA, a known hormone disruptor

The conclusion? Dig out your Boy Scout canteen. Stainless steel, glass, and ceramic containers are the safest. While it isn't practical to carry a glass bottle on your power walk, more and more stores are carrying light stainless steel bottles. They are dishwasher safe, eliminating harmful bacteria build up, and are BPA-free.

Recipes That Help You Drink More Water

Plain water is uninspiring. Flavored waters are everywhere, but watch out for hidden calories. To be sure you know what you are drinking, try these fantastic, nutritious recipes.

Raspberry "Soda"

SERVES 4

100 calories
1 g fat
24 g carbohydrates
2 g protein
100 mg sodium
8 g fiber

INGREDIENTS
2 pints raspberries
2 tablespoons honey
Juice of 1 lime
2 quarts seltzer water

This soda can be made with any seasonal fruit. Try it with peaches, pineapples, pomegranates, and even orange or apple juice. It's the bubbles that make it fun.

Combine berries and honey in a small saucepan over high heat. Cook until juicy and bubbly, about 5 minutes. Cool slightly, transfer to a blender, and puree until smooth. Strain into a pitcher and add seltzer. Pour over ice to serve.

Spa Water

The spa is where you go to get refreshed and rejuvenated. You can replicate the experience in your own kitchen with this herb-infused water. Make it in the morning, and let it steep all day so it's ready when you get home from work.

Combine lemon and gently crushed herbs in a large pitcher. Add water, stir, and steep for 1–8 hours. Strain over ice to serve.

SERVES 4

25 calories
< 1 g fat
5 g carbohydrates
1 g protein
10 mg sodium
2 g fiber

INGREDIENTS
1 small lemon, sliced in wheels
1 cup fresh spearmint leaves
½ cup fresh rosemary needles
½ cup fresh tarragon
2 quarts water

Green Ginger Tea

You can also try this recipe with jasmine or lemon herbal tea. Be sure to pick the decaffeinated tea, or you'll defeat the purpose, as caffeine is a diuretic.

Combine tea bags, ginger, honey, and lime in a large, heat-proof bowl. Add boiling water and steep for 15 minutes. Strain into a large pitcher and add cold water. Serve over ice.

SERVES 4

35 calories
0 g fat
10 g carbohydrates
0 g protein
0 mg sodium
0 g fiber

INGREDIENTS
2 green tea bags (decaffeinated)
1 knuckle of fresh ginger root, sliced thin
2 tablespoons honey
Juice of 1 lime
2 cups boiling water
2 quarts cold water

Aguas Frescas

SERVES 8

130 calories
0 g fat
36 g carbohydrates
1 g protein
5 mg sodium
< 1 g fiber

INGREDIENTS
*1 cup tamarind pulp, or 20
    tamarind pods, peeled
¾ cup honey
2–3 quarts water*

Aguas frescas are cool, refreshing beverages served on every street corner in Mexico. They are made from fruit, herbs, rice, and spices, as well as tangy tamarind.

1. Combine tamarind and honey in a large, heat-proof bowl. Boil 1 quart of water, pour into bowl, and steep until cool.

2. Remove tamarind seeds, transfer to a blender, and process until smooth. Strain into a pitcher and add remaining water. Serve over ice.

Tamarind
Tamarind is a sticky brown pulp found inside a fuzzy brown bean pod from a tropical evergreen tree. The tart pulp is as popular worldwide as lemons are in the West. Purchase tamarind pods whole at Asian or Mexican markets, or find the pulp in brick form, with or without seeds.

Melon Cooler

SERVES 4

70 calories
0 g fat
18 g carbohydrates
2 g protein
35 mg sodium
2 g fiber

INGREDIENTS
*1 cantaloupe, diced
Juice of 1 lemon
½ cup fresh mint
2 quarts water*

Try this recipe with any melon, including honeydew or watermelon! Be sure to let it chill at least an hour for maximum refreshment.

Working in batches, combine melon, lemon, and mint in a blender, and process with water as needed until smooth. Strain into a large pitcher, add remaining water, and chill. Serve over ice.

Tropical Punch

You can add any number of tropical fruits to this recipe.
Try guava, passion fruit, papaya, or kiwis.

Combine mango, pineapple, banana, orange juice, coconut milk, and lime juice in a blender. Puree until smooth. Strain into a large pitcher. Add remaining water, stir, and serve over ice.

SERVES 8

120 calories
4.5 g fat
21 g carbohydrates
1 g protein
10 mg sodium
2 g fiber

INGREDIENTS
1 mango, peeled and diced
2 cups pineapple chunks
1 banana
1 cup orange juice
1 (5.6-ounce) can coconut milk
Juice of 1 lime
2 quarts water

Iced Hibiscus

The dried hibiscus flower turns this infusion a brilliant red.
Its flavor is slightly tangy, and oh-so-refreshing.

In a large saucepan, combine hibiscus, cinnamon stick, star anise, honey, lime, and 2 cups water. Bring to a boil, remove from heat, and steep 15 minutes. Strain into a large pitcher, add remaining water, and chill. Serve over ice.

SERVES 6

30 calories
0 g fat
8 g carbohydrates
0 g protein
0 mg sodium
< 1 g fiber

INGREDIENTS
¼ cup dried hibiscus flower (also called Jamaican sorrel)
1 cinnamon stick
2 or 3 star anise
2 tablespoons honey
Juice of 1 lime
2 quarts water

Chapter 21

Food for the Active Family

Following dietary guidelines is important for everyone. But if you're extremely active, you need extra attention. Athletes young and old should pay special attention to their nutritional needs.

The Power of Carbohydrates

Carbohydrates are the most important fuel food for athletes. Regardless of the sport, carbohydrates are the body's preferred source of energy. They are broken down into simple sugars, absorbed, and converted into energy to fuel muscle contractions.

Glucose that is not needed immediately is stored in muscle tissue and the liver in the form of glycogen. Most exercise relies on stored glycogen for energy, especially when short bursts of energy are needed, as in weight lifting or in the stop-and-go sprinting of racket sports. During longer endurance sports, the body uses fat as energy, but it relies on glycogen to convert the fat into something the muscles can use.

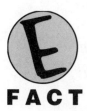

FACT

The body can store around 2,000 carbohydrate calories. When glycogen stores are full, the excess carbohydrates are stored as fat. If not enough carbohydrates are eaten, protein from muscle and other tissues will be tapped as an energy source, which can damage the body's ability to build and maintain tissue.

Depletion of glycogen stores, through prolonged exercise, or an inadequate diet, results in the dreaded "bonk," also known as "hitting the wall." The body runs out of fuel for immediate exercise. This typically occurs after sixty to ninety minutes of vigorous activity, depending on the conditioning of the athlete. To avoid this, athletes try to increase glycogen stores before exercising, replenish during the activity, and refill afterward to prepare for the next workout.

Simple sugars are the easiest form of carbohydrates for the body to absorb. Because they convert quickly to energy, they are an essential element of sports drinks. (The speed with which they are converted can be experienced in the dreaded "sugar high.") Complex carbohydrates take longer to absorb, and therefore fuel the body at a slower rate. To increase glycogen stores, complex carbohydrates from starch are preferred. Foods like potatoes, pasta, whole grains, and cereals are an important element in the athlete's diet.

Food as Fuel

Athletes are keenly aware of the fuel aspect of food, especially when it's running out. And they are familiar with the instant rejuvenation a little fuel can give when they're running on empty.

Pre-Exercise: Food That Gets You Going

Eating before an exercise routine is essential, but it should be planned carefully. Too much food too close to the activity can give you nausea, cramps, or worse. The sloshing feeling in your stomach can also be distracting. It's best to give your food time to digest.

The best pre-exercise eating plan begins two to three hours prior to the activity. A light meal high in complex carbohydrates and some protein is ideal. A bowl of cereal, a peanut butter sandwich, a baked potato with cottage cheese, or a bagel are all good choices. Avoid fat, because it is hard to digest, and it stays in the stomach longer.

Thirty to sixty minutes prior to your workout have a piece of fruit or an energy bar. These last-minute carbohydrates can help boost energy to get you started. Some athletes take a bite of simple sugar foods just before heading out the door. Experiment with this, because some people cannot handle the spike and dip in blood glucose during their sport.

So, how much food do you actually need for your workout?

- Calorie needs for training vary, but they generally hover around 17–20 calories per pound for maintenance, and 16–17 calories per pound to lose body fat.
- Protein needs for training range between 0.5 and 0.6 grams per pound. Carbohydrate needs for training are 3–5 grams per pound, and more for higher-intensity endurance sports.
- Fat needs for training are about 0.5 grams per pound, or the balance of your calories after protein and carbohydrates.
- Fluid needs for training vary too, but are generally 1 quart (32 ounces) for every 1,000 calories, plus additional fluid for exercise, from 2–5 quarts depending on the intensity.

Caffeine before exercise is not recommended. It is a diuretic, which can cause dehydration. It can also cause nausea, muscle tremors, or headaches. The effects depend on your personal habits, and your level of addiction.

During Exercise: Electrolytes and Carbs

The electrolytes sodium and potassium are salts that can carry an electrical charge. Cells rely on them to carry impulses for muscles and nerves. You get plenty of electrolytes in your food, so regular daily exercise does not require electrolyte replacement. But with constant, vigorous activity for over an hour, as in long-distance running, electrolyte replacement can be beneficial.

The sports drink phenomenon of today all began in the 1960s with a football coach at the University of Florida. He was concerned that his athletes ran out of energy during practices. University doctors came up with a beverage that combines sodium, potassium, and carbohydrate with water to combat the loss of vital fluid in the Florida heat. The drink was a success, and soon teams from all over the country were ordering the Florida Gator's drink. Today, it is on the sidelines of every major sporting event as Gatorade.

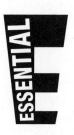

Endurance athletes need more than the boost they get from a sports drink. Carbohydrate gels, candy, and even soda pop are common midevent glucose boosters. The burst of energy they provide helps delay the "bonk." Elite athletes will sometimes pop a glucose pill close to the finish line for an extra edge.

Sports drinks are everywhere, and they are marketed relentlessly. But there is no reason to consume this high-calorie, high-sodium drink on a regular basis. It is certainly not something to drink simply to quench thirst.

If you are a serious athlete, sip a sports drink every fifteen to thirty minutes throughout your activity to maintain a constant energy level. Look for a sport drink with less fructose. This sugar causes bloating and cramping in some, and can delay water absorption, which makes exercise feel harder.

After Exercise: Food for Recuperation

Exercise takes its toll on the body. Athletes are often injured, and the body's motions wear away at joints, bones, connective tissues, and muscles. Proper nutrition is vital to immediate recovery from exercise as well as long-term strength and stamina.

After exercise, fluid is the first thing your body wants and needs. Drink twenty to twenty-four ounces for every pound lost during your exercise session (this requires you weighing yourself before and after). Within the first fifteen minutes after exercise, get some carbohydrate to begin restoring glycogen. A glass of orange juice is perfect.

Muscle glycogen synthesis, the conversion of carbohydrate to glycogen for your muscles, is greater immediately after exercise, and for about forty-five minutes. Within that time frame you should consume 100–200 grams of carbohydrates. This immediately begins to rebuild your glycogen stores for later. After two hours your body's ability to convert carbohydrate to glycogen is reduced by 50 percent.

Protein is also needed after exercise to begin rebuilding muscle tissue damaged by the wear and tear of your sport. In addition, protein helps improve water absorption, which improves muscle hydration. Consume twenty-five to fifty grams of protein within the forty-five-minute window.

This 4:1 ratio of carbohydrates to protein, plus water, is easier to digest, and faster to absorb, when taken in liquid form. Smoothies and specially formulated sports drinks are ideal. See the recipes at the end of this chapter for a few ideas.

Sport Food Myths

There is a lot of sports nutrition information out there, and much of it is sound. But often, what you hear in the locker room is less reliable. Here are a few commonly held beliefs that are no longer considered valid.

Myth: Eating More Protein Speeds Muscle Building and Builds Strength

While amino acids do build muscle, and athletes should eat more protein, it is not possible to build muscle or strength by eating more protein. Your body will burn what it needs for energy and store the rest as fat.

Myth: Athletes Need More Vitamins for Energy

Vitamins do not provide energy; calories do. Vitamins are in the food you eat. Athletes need the same amount of vitamins as everyone else.

Myth: Athletes Need Extra Sodium and Potassium to Replace Sweat Loss

Only in extreme physical exertion do athletes lose sodium and potassium. In regular exercise it is only necessary to take in fluid, which helps keep the salts in balance.

Myth: Skipping Breakfast Helps Burn More Fat

Skipping a meal will result in fewer calories burned overall. That's because you will get tired faster and won't be working at your usual potential.

Myth: Carb Loading the Night Before an Activity Gives You More Energy

Carbohydrate loading is intended as part of a long process of building glycogen stores. It should be ongoing throughout the athlete's training, which includes the "taper," a reduction of exertion paired with an increase in carbohydrate intake during the last week before a big event.

Supplements

There are hundreds of products on the market claiming to improve performance. Sports supplements are known as ergogenic aids, from the Greek *ergon*, meaning "potential for work." They include vitamins, synthetic drugs, and hormones, all believed to build muscle mass, strength, and stamina. These products are not regulated by the FDA, and not all have been properly tested.

Sports supplements are required to list all ingredients on their labels, but if a consumer is unfamiliar with harmful substances, the list will be meaningless. Beware when a product claims "rapid results," cites oversimplified research, or provides statistics from only one study. Look for "IOC approved" on the label, which is a thumbs-up from the International Olympic Committee.

The following harmful ergogenic aids are banned by the IOC.

Anabolic Steroids

These steroids are similar to the male hormone testosterone and are taken to build muscle mass. Side effects include high blood pressure, heart disease, liver damage, stroke, blood clots, depression, and aggression. In males they create baldness, acne, infertility, breast enlargement, and erectile dysfunction. In females they create a deeper voice, smaller breasts, facial and body hair, and menstrual irregularities.

Natural Steroids

Androstenedione and dehydroepiandrosterone are actually prohormones. They are not testosterone, but break down into testosterone in the body. The effects are similar to anabolic steroids, creating a hormone imbalance. These products, if taken too young, stunt growth by tricking the body into believing it has already gone through puberty.

Creatine

Manufactured by your body naturally in the liver and pancreas, creatine supplements are taken to increase strength. Use can lead to muscle cramps and tears, weight gain, diarrhea, abdominal pain, dehydration, seizures, and kidney failure.

Ephedra

This herb, also known as ephedrine or ma huang, is taken as a fat burner. It raises body temperature and speeds the nervous system, increasing metabolism. It also creates anxiety, insomnia, heart problems, stroke, and in some cases, death.

Recipes for Before and After Exercise

Forget the protein bars and sports drinks. What your body wants is real food, preferably made especially for it, by you.

Muesli

*Muesli means "mixture," and it began as a health food developed
by Swiss physicians in the 1800s. Today it is a breakfast staple
around the world. Mixtures vary, as does soaking time. The
longer the soak, the softer the oats become.*

Combine oats, raisins, honey, and milk in a bowl and refrigerate for 30
minutes, or overnight for softer oats. Before serving, stir in almonds, yogurt,
apple, and sesame seeds.

SERVES 2

210 calories
9 g fat
85 g carbohydrates
18 g protein
150 mg sodium
8 g fiber

INGREDIENTS

½ cup rolled oats
½ cup raisins
1 tablespoon honey
2 cups fat-free milk
¼ cup sliced almonds
¼ cup nonfat yogurt
1 apple, grated
1 teaspoon sesame seeds

Tuna Wraps

*Capers add a distinctive salty tang to any recipe. They are small
buds from an evergreen shrub that have been pickled in salty, vin-
egary brine. Find them in the market near the pickles and olives.*

In a large bowl, combine tuna, mayonnaise, mustard, celery, onion, and
capers. Divide evenly between four tortillas, and top each with shredded
lettuce. Fold the side edges toward the center, then roll up from the bottom.
Serve as is or cut in half.

SERVES 4

300 calories
15 g fat
25 g carbohydrates
15 g protein
690 mg sodium
3 g fiber

INGREDIENTS

1 (6-ounce) can water-packed
    tuna
¼ cup mayonnaise
1 tablespoon Dijon mustard
1 stalk celery, diced
2 tablespoons diced onion
1 tablespoon capers
4 large whole-wheat tortillas
2 cups shredded lettuce

Banana Bran Muffins

Bran is pure plant fiber, or cellulose. Paired with whole-wheat flour, wheat germ, and oat bran, these muffins are a powerhouse of complex carbohydrates. Fold in dried fruits, such as dates, figs, cranberries, or apricots for an additional burst of chewy sweetness and nutrition.

1. Preheat oven to 375°F. Coat muffin pan with pan spray and line with paper cups.

2. Beat together eggs, oil, honey, molasses, vanilla, buttermilk, and banana and set aside.

3. In a separate bowl, stir together flour, germ, brans, baking powder, baking soda, salt, and spices.

4. Pour the egg mixture into the flour mixture and stir together until just incorporated.

5. Fill muffin cups to the rim with muffin batter. Bake until risen and golden brown, about 20 minutes. A toothpick inserted into the middle muffin should come out clean. Cool 15 minutes before removing. Store airtight at room temperature for 2 days, or freeze for up to 2 weeks.

MAKES 1 DOZEN MUFFINS

per muffin
270 calories
9 g fat
43 g carbohydrates
10 g protein
390 mg sodium
9 g fiber

INGREDIENTS
2 eggs
⅓ cup canola oil
⅓ cup honey
⅓ cup molasses
1 tablespoon vanilla extract
1⅓ cups buttermilk
2 ripe bananas, sliced
1 cup whole-wheat flour
1 cup wheat germ
2 cups wheat bran
1 cup oat bran
1 teaspoon baking powder
2 teaspoons baking soda
½ teaspoon kosher salt
1 teaspoon ground ginger
1 teaspoon ground cinnamon
1 teaspoon ground nutmeg

Braised Moroccan Beans

SERVES 6

350 calories
10 g fat
59 g carbohydrates
11 g protein
660 mg sodium
10 g fiber

INGREDIENTS
2 tablespoons olive oil
1 yellow onion, diced
4 cloves garlic
1 teaspoon ground cumin
1 teaspoon ground coriander
1 large carrot, diced
2 stalks celery, diced
6 new potatoes, halved
1 (15-ounce) can chickpeas
1 (15-ounce) can lima beans
2–4 cups water
Juice of 1 lemon
½ cup sliced almonds
1 cup raisins
½ cup fresh cilantro, chopped

Moroccan stews like this one are classically cooked in a conical casserole dish called a tagine, *but any old casserole dish will do. Serve with brown rice or couscous, a fine-grained pasta.*

1. Preheat oven to 350°F.

2. Heat oil in a large sauté pan over high heat. Add onions and garlic and sauté until tender.

3. Add spices, carrot, and celery and continue cooking until translucent.

4. Transfer to a casserole dish and add potatoes, chickpeas, lima beans, and water to cover.

5. Cover and bake until bubbly and tender, about 45 minutes. Stir in lemon juice, almonds, raisins, and top with cilantro before serving.

Recovery Smoothie

If kept chilled and clean, eggs are perfectly safe to eat raw. If you are uneasy, substitute 1 scoop of protein powder. Choose whey protein, which is more easily absorbed by the body than soy protein.

Combine banana, strawberry, yolks, oats, wheat germ, milk, and yogurt in a blender. Puree until smooth, add ice, and puree again. Serve immediately.

SERVES 2

530 calories
12 g fat
81 g carbohydrates
26 g protein
160 mg sodium
12 g fiber

INGREDIENTS
1 banana
1 cup strawberries
3 egg yolks
1 cup rolled oats
¼ cup wheat germ
2 cups fat-free milk
¼ cup nonfat plain yogurt
2–3 cups ice

Power Water

This homemade sports drink has good carbohydrates and electrolytes, and it tastes better than anything you can buy at the store.

In a large pitcher combine tea bag, sugar, salt, orange juice, and boiling water. Steep 15 minutes. Remove tea bag, stir in remaining water, fill your sports bottle, and chill.

SERVES 4

30 calories
0 g fat
8 g carbohydrates
0 g protein
150 mg sodium
0 g fiber

INGREDIENTS
1 lemon tea bag
2 tablespoons sugar
¼ teaspoon kosher salt
¼ cup orange juice
2 cups boiling water
4 cups ice water

Homemade Energy Bars

MAKES 15 BARS

240 calories
12 g fat
30 g carbohydrates
5 g protein
130 mg sodium
4 g fiber

INGREDIENTS
2 cups rolled oats
½ cup raisins
½ cup dried figs
½ cup walnuts
*¼ cup unsalted hulled
    sunflower seeds*
¾ cup whole-wheat flour
1 teaspoon cinnamon
1 teaspoon baking soda
¼ teaspoon kosher salt
½ cup vegetable oil
½ cup date sugar
1 egg
*1 cup unsweetened
    applesauce*
2 teaspoons vanilla

*These bars are much tastier than the store-bought variety. Store
them airtight for 2–3 days, or freeze them for up to two weeks.
They make a great midafternoon pick-me-up snack.*

1. Preheat oven to 350°F. Coat a 9" × 13" baking pan with pan spray.

2. In a large bowl, combine the oats, raisins, figs, walnuts, sunflower seeds, flour, cinnamon, baking soda, and salt.

3. In a separate bowl stir together oil, date sugar, egg, apple sauce, and vanilla.

4. Pour wet ingredients into dry ingredients and mix thoroughly. Transfer batter to prepared pan and bake until golden brown, about 35–40 minutes. Cool 10 minutes, then cut into bars.

Appendix A
A Week of Menu Ideas

Monday

Breakfast	Blueberry Bran Muffins with Orange Marmalade, Orange Juice	page 285
Lunch	Egg Salad Cracker Canapés, Honey Lemon Iced Tea	page 285
Snack	Mom's Trail Mix and Cinnamon Milk	page 286
Dinner	Mixed Green Salad, Turkey Burgers, Whole-Grain Oatmeal Spice Cookies	page 286

Tuesday

Breakfast	High-Fiber Coconut-Mango Smoothies	page 286
Lunch	Whole-Wheat Veggie Wraps with Sesame Rice Vinaigrette	page 287
Snack	Gingered Plums and Asian Pears, Kafir Limeade	page 287
Dinner	Egg Fried Rice, Vegetable Stir-Fry, Toasted Honey Almonds	page 287–288

Wednesday

Breakfast	Muesli, Pomegranate Juice	page 288
Lunch	Chopped Chicken Waldorf Salad	page 288
Snack	Red Yam Dip with Multigrain Bread Sticks, Cantaloupe Cooler	page 288–289
Dinner	Almond Quinoa Salad, Foil-Baked Salmon, Pink Grapefruit Jellied Salad	page 289

Thursday

Breakfast	Whole-Grain Sesame Banana Bread, Spiced Herbal Tea	page 290
Lunch	Cucumber-Chickpea Salad with Minted Yogurt Dressing	page 290
Snack	Pita Chips, Mint Spritzer	page 290
Dinner	Tabouli, Braised Lamb, Fresh Seasonal Fruit	page 291

Friday

Breakfast	Red Blast Vitamin Smoothie, Whole-Wheat Cinnamon Toast with Berry Preserves	page 291
Lunch	Southwestern Five-Bean Salad with Whole-Grain Cumin Crackers	page 291–292
Snack	Coconut Popcorn, Horchata	page 292
Dinner	Fish Tacos, Fruit Skewers with Lime	page 292

Saturday

Breakfast	Frittata with Wild Mushrooms	page 292
Lunch	Whole Grain Focaccia with Grilled Vegetables	page 293
Snack	Apricot and Fig Granola Bars, Almond Milk	page 293
Dinner	Caprese Salad, Pasta Primavera with Parmesan Chicken, Espresso Granita	page 293–294

Sunday

Breakfast	Breakfast-Granola Parfait	page 294
Lunch	Grilled Tuna Niçoise	page 294
Snack	Whole-Wheat Baguette with Roquefort Spread, Spa Water	page 295
Dinner	Celery Root Remoulade, Dijon-Marinated Grilled Chicken, Whole-Wheat Orange Crepes	page 295–296

Monday

Breakfast

Blueberry Bran Muffins

See recipe for Banana Bran Muffins in Chapter 21. Replace bananas with 1½ cups fresh or frozen blueberries.

Lunch

Egg Salad Cracker Canapés

Egg salad is a simple dish. But presented on crackers it has new dignity. If you want to really impress, serve these on a silver platter.

1. Place eggs in small saucepan and cover with water. Boil over high heat for 5 minutes. Turn off heat and let sit in the hot water 20 minutes. Transfer to a bowl of ice water and chill for 10 minutes.

2. Peel the cooled eggs, then chop fine. Combine in a large bowl with mayonnaise, mustard, onion powder, celery, radishes, and pepper. Spoon a teaspoon of egg salad onto each cracker and top with chopped parsley or a sprinkle of paprika, and serve.

Honey Lemon Iced Tea

Try adding a few sprigs of fresh thyme to this recipe for a subtle touch of summertime.

Combine tea bags, honey, and lemon juice in a large, heat-proof bowl. Add boiling water and steep for 15 minutes. Strain into a large pitcher and add cold water. Serve over ice.

Egg Salad Cracker Canapés
MAKES ABOUT 2 DOZEN

INGREDIENTS
4 eggs
1 tablespoon mayonnaise
1 tablespoon Dijon mustard
½ teaspoon powdered onion
1 stalk celery, chopped fine
3 radishes, minced
½ teaspoon ground black pepper
Whole-wheat crackers
2–3 tablespoons chopped
    parsley
Paprika for dusting

Honey Lemon Iced Tea
SERVES 4–6

INGREDIENTS
2 lemon herb teabags
2 tablespoons honey
Juice of 2 lemons
2 cups boiling water
2 quarts cold water

Snack

Mom's Trail Mix

See recipe, Chapter 15.

Cinnamon Milk

This milk is a welcome change from hot cocoa, and it's just as tasty. Try it iced.

Combine milk and cinnamon in a large saucepan and bring to a boil over high heat. Reduce heat to low and simmer 15 minutes. Remove from heat, stir in honey and vanilla, and serve. Or cool, and serve over ice.

Dinner

Mixed Green Salad

See recipe, Chapter 17.

Turkey Burgers

See recipe, Chapter 6.

Whole-Grain Oatmeal Spice Cookies

See Carob Chip Oatmeal Cookie recipe, Chapter 9. Omit carob chips and fold in 1 teaspoon cinnamon, 1 teaspoon nutmeg, 1 teaspoon ginger, ¼ teaspoon ground cloves, and 1½ cups golden raisins. Bake as directed.

Tuesday

Breakfast

High Fiber Coconut-Mango Smoothies

You can add any number of tropical fruits to this smoothie. Bananas make it a little sweeter, pineapple a little more tart.

Combine mango, coconut milk, oat bran, wheat germ, coconut, milk, and agave syrup. Puree until smooth, add ice, and puree again. Serve immediately.

Lunch

Whole-Wheat Veggie Wraps with Sesame Rice Vinaigrette

This is a deliciously fresh way to get your veggies.

1. In a large bowl whisk together peanut and sesame oil, garlic, ginger, rice vinegar, honey, soy sauce, and lime juice. Add carrots, celery, zucchini, green onions, bean sprouts, sesame seeds, and cilantro. Toss well to thoroughly coat.

2. Divide salad evenly between each tortilla. Fold sides of tortilla toward the center, then roll up from the bottom. Serve as is, or cut in half, on the bias.

Snack

Gingered Plums and Asian Pears

Asian pears and plums have a short season in the late summer, but you can enjoy a variation of this recipe all year long. Try peaches and cherries, oranges and strawberries, or bananas and kiwi.

In a large bowl, whisk together orange juice, honey, and ginger. Add fruit, toss to coat, then set aside to macerate for 30–60 minutes before serving.

Kaffir Limeade

The Kaffir lime tree produces a fruit, but its fruit is not as popular as its unique double-lobed, figure-8 leaf. The leaf's intense aroma is an essential ingredient throughout Southeast Asia. Look for Kaffir lime leaves in Asian markets. If you have trouble finding them, you can substitute the grated zest of 4–5 limes.

Combine leaves and honey in a large heat-proof bowl. Add boiling water and steep 30 minutes. Strain into a large pitcher, add cold water, and chill. Serve over ice.

Dinner

Egg Fried Rice
See recipe, Chapter 6.

Whole-Wheat Veggie Wraps with Sesame Rice Vinaigrette
SERVES 4

INGREDIENTS
1 teaspoon peanut oil
1 teaspoon sesame oil
1 clove garlic, sliced
2 teaspoons ginger root, grated
1 teaspoon rice vinegar
1 teaspoon honey
3 teaspoons soy sauce
Juice of 2 limes (about 1 tablespoon)
2 medium carrots, grated
2 stalks celery, sliced thin
1 zucchini, grated
1 cup green onions, chopped
1 cup bean sprouts
2 tablespoons sesame seeds
½ cup cilantro, chopped
4 large whole-wheat tortillas

Gingered Plums and Asian Pears
SERVES 4

INGREDIENTS
1 cup orange juice
1 tablespoon honey
1 tablespoon grated ginger
2 ripe plums, sliced
2 Asian pears, sliced

Kaffir Limeade
SERVES 6-8

INGREDIENTS
6–8 Kaffir lime leaves, gently bruised
¼ cup honey
1 quart boiling water
1 quart cold water

Vegetable Stir-Fry

See Chicken Stir-Fry recipe, Chapter 17. Replace chicken with a mixture of chopped vegetables, including squash, cabbage, peas, spinach, red onion, carrots, bean sprouts, water chestnuts, and bamboo shoots. Cook as directed.

Toasted Honey Almonds

If you like things on the spicy side, add a pinch or two of cayenne pepper.

Preheat oven to 375°F. Spread nuts on baking sheet in an even layer. Toast until fragrant and browned, 10–15 minutes. While hot, toss nuts in olive oil and honey, and spread out again to cool. Store airtight in the refrigerator or freezer.

Wednesday

Breakfast

Muesli

See recipe, Chapter 21.

Lunch

Chopped Chicken Waldorf Salad

See Waldorf Salad recipe, Chapter 10. Add 3 cups cooked, diced chicken. Prepare as directed.

Snack

Sweet Potato Dip

See Red Yam Spread recipe, Chapter 8. Replace yams with yellow sweet potatoes. Cook as directed, then add an extra ¼–½ cup water while blending to create a thinner, dressing-like consistency.

Multigrain Bread Sticks

See Multigrain Cracker recipe, Chapter 7. Make dough as directed. Rather than roll into flat crackers, cut dough into long, thin strips. Bake as directed.

Cantaloupe Cooler

See Melon Cooler recipe, Chapter 20. Add an extra cup or two of cantaloupe to give this refresher a burst of melon.

Dinner

Almond Quinoa Salad

You can stir in more herbs, or add some crunchy vegetables. This dish also tastes great warm.

In a large sauté pan over high heat, cook onions, celery, and garlic in olive oil until tender. Add thyme and quinoa and cook 5–10 minutes, stirring, until toasted and brown. Add water and bring to a boil. Reduce heat to low, cover, and cook 15 minutes, until liquid is absorbed. Remove from heat, fluff with a fork, and cool. Just before serving, stir in lemon juice and almonds.

Foil-Baked Salmon

See recipe, Chapter 17.

Pink Grapefruit Jellied Salad

In addition to dessert, try serving this refreshing, jiggly treat as a salad. Place wedges on a lettuce leaf, topped with a dollop of cottage cheese.

1. In a large bowl, dissolve the lime and lemon gelatin in the boiling water. Add the cold water, and chill until partially set, about 30 minutes.

2. Meanwhile combine the lemon juice, grapefruit, and pineapple, and stir into partially set gelatin. Pour into a mold and chill for at least 6 hours, or overnight.

3. Unmold the set salad by dipping the bottom of the mold briefly into hot tap water (about 5 seconds). Turn it out onto a platter, tap once or twice, and lift up the mold.

Almond Quinoa Salad
SERVES 4–6

INGREDIENTS
2 tablespoons olive oil
1 large yellow onion, chopped
1 stalk celery, chopped
3 cloves garlic, minced
1 tablespoon fresh thyme, chopped
2 cups quinoa
4 cups water
Juice of 1 lemon
1 cup sliced almond

Pink Grapefruit Jelllied Salad
SERVES 6

INGREDIENTS
1 (3-ounce) package sugar-free lime gelatin
1 (3-ounce) package sugar-free lemon gelatin
2 cups boiling water
1½ cups cold water
3 tablespoons lemon juice
2 pink grapefruits, peeled and diced
1 (8-ounce) can crushed pineapple, drained

Thursday

Breakfast

Whole-Grain Sesame Banana Bread

See Banana Walnut Bread recipe, Chapter 9. Omit walnuts, and replace them with 2 tablespoons toasted sesame seeds. Bake as directed.

Spiced Herbal Tea

This tea is fantastic hot or cold. It also makes a delicious poaching liquid for apples or pears. Simmer the fruit until tender, then strain the liquid and serve it in steamy mugs on the side.

Combine tea, spices, and honey in a large saucepan. Add water and bring to a boil. Reduce heat and simmer 10 minutes. Remove from heat, strain into a heat-proof pitcher and serve.

Lunch

Cucumber-Chickpea Salad with Minted Yogurt Dressing

This salad is similar to Indian raita, a cool tangy salad that relieves the palate during a spicy meal of curries.

In a large bowl, mix together yogurt, cumin, mint, and salt. Add cucumbers, onions, chickpeas, and refrigerate for 1–2 hours to allow flavors to mingle. Serve chilled.

Snack

Pita Chips

See recipe, Chapter 16.

Mint Spritzer

Spearmint is the most common mint in the supermarkets, but if you can find peppermint, try it here. The flavor is, well, pepperier.

Combine mint, honey, and lemon juice in large pitcher, add seltzer, and chill for 1–2 hours. Strain and serve over ice.

Dinner

Tabouli
See recipe, Chapter 10.

Braised Lamb
See Venison Stew, Chapter 6. Replace venison with cubed lamb shoulder, and add 3–4 extra cloves of garlic. Cook as directed.

Fresh Seasonal Fruit

Friday

Breakfast

Red Blast Vitamin Smoothie
This tangy smoothie will really wake you up in the morning. To roast the beet, wrap it in foil and bake at 500°F for 30–45 minutes, until tender. You can also microwave it, as you would a potato, until tender.

Combine beat, strawberries, raspberries, cranberries, wheat germ, and pomegranate juice in a blender, and puree until smooth and liquefied. Add yogurt, honey, and ice; puree again; and serve.

Lunch

Southwestern Five-Bean Salad
This salad tastes best if it can marinate for a few hours. Make it in the morning and let it chill all day.

In a large bowl, combine the honey, oil, lime, and pepper and mix well to combine. Add bell pepper, chilies, cilantro, cumin, chili powder, beans, onions, and corn. Toss well to coat, cover with plastic wrap, and refrigerate for 2 hours, or overnight.

Red Blast Vitamin Smoothies
SERVES 2

INGREDIENTS
1 large beet, roasted
1 cup strawberries
1 cup raspberries
1 cup fresh or frozen cranberries
¼ cup wheat germ
1 cup pomegranate juice
1 cup yogurt
½ cup honey
2–3 cups ice

Southwestern Five-Bean Salad
SERVES 4

INGREDIENTS
½ cup honey
⅓ cup canola oil
½ cup lime juice
½ teaspoon ground black pepper
1 red bell pepper, chopped
1 (4-ounce) can of chopped green chilies
1 cup chopped cilantro
1 tablespoon ground cumin
1 teaspoon chili powder
1 (15-ounce) can kidney beans, drained
1 (15-ounce) can yellow wax beans, drained
1 (15-ounce) can green string beans, drained
1 (15-ounce) can black beans, drained and rinsed
1 (15-ounce) can navy beans, drained
1 small purple onion, chopped and soaked in cold water for 15–20 minutes
2 scallions, chopped
1 (15-ounce) can corn, drained

Whole-Grain Cumin Crackers

See Multigrain Crackers recipe, Chapter 7. Add to the dough 2 tablespoons of toasted whole cumin seeds. Using a dry skillet over medium heat, toast spices, shaking the pan, until they are golden and fragrant, about 2–3 minutes. Cool, and crush in a mortar or grind in a coffee mill, then add to the dough before kneading. Bake as directed.

Snack

Coconut Popcorn

See Cheesy Popcorn recipe, Chapter 15. Omit Parmesan cheese and replace it with 1 cup of unsweetened, shredded coconut, and 1 tablespoon date sugar.

Horchata

See recipe, Chapter 6.

Dinner

Fish Tacos

See Soft Taco recipe in Chapter 17. Replace steak with any grilled seafood, such as cod, trout, salmon, or tuna.

Fruit Skewers with Lime

See Fruit Kebab recipe, Chapter 15. Use tropical fruits, including pineapple, papaya, mango, and kiwi. Omit yogurt dip, and serve with lime wedges and a shaker of chili powder.

Saturday

Breakfast

Frittata with Wild Mushrooms

See Spinach and Mushroom Frittata, Chapter 6. Omit the spinach and replace it with 3 cups of sliced assorted wild mushrooms. Choose fresh mushrooms or reconstitute dried mushrooms. Soak dried mushrooms in warm water for

30 minutes, until tender. (Reserve mushroom liquid for vegetable soup or use it to make a delicious rice pilaf.)

Lunch

Whole-Grain Focaccia with Grilled Vegetables

This is just one example of the versatility of yeast dough. Focaccia is traditionally a thick bread, lightly topped with minimal ingredients. In the United States it is used more as sandwich bread. Here it is getting dangerously, but deliciously, close to pizza.

Preheat oven to 450°F. After dough is risen, divide in two and shape into round, flat discs. Place on a baking sheet coated with pan spray, and rub with olive oil. Coat vegetables lightly in oil, and grill, or broil, until browned. Place vegetables on top of dough, sprinkle with cheese and herbs, and bake until golden brown, about 20–30 minutes.

Snack

Apricot and Fig Granola Bars

Personalize these bars with your favorite fruits, nuts, and spices.

1. Preheat oven to 325°F. Coat a 9" × 13" baking dish with pan spray. In a large bowl, stir together oats, sunflower seeds, flour, fruit, walnuts, date sugar, salt, and baking soda. Add oil, honey, and vanilla, and mix well to moisten.

2. Press mixture into prepared pan, and bake 20 minutes, until golden brown. Cool 10 minutes before slicing into bars.

Dinner

Caprese Salad

See recipe, Chapter 17.

Whole-Grain Focaccia with Grilled Vegetables
SERVES 4–6

INGREDIENTS
1 recipe Multigrain Bread, Chapter 10
2–3 tablespoons olive oil
3–4 cups assorted vegetables, such as squash, eggplant, tomatoes, and onions, sliced thin
½ cup Parmesan cheese
2 tablespoons Italian Blend, Chapter 12

Apricot and Fig Granola Bars
MAKES 10–12 BARS

INGREDIENTS
4½ cups rolled oats
¼ cup sunflower seeds
1 cup whole-wheat flour
½ cup dried apricots, chopped
½ cup dried figs, chopped
1 cup walnuts
⅓ cup date sugar
½ teaspoon kosher salt
1 teaspoon baking soda
⅔ cup canola oil
½ cup honey
1 teaspoon vanilla extract

Pasta Primavera with Parmesan Chicken

See Pasta Primavera recipe, Chapter 17. When sautéing garlic after pasta has been cooked, also sauté 12 boneless, skinless chicken breasts, sliced into ½-inch strips, until browned and cooked through. Add to pasta with vegetables.

Espresso Granita

Serve this refreshing summer dessert in chilled glasses so it doesn't melt too soon.

Combine ingredients in a shallow baking dish and place in the freezer. Use a fork to mix up ice crystals every 20 minutes until the entire pan is frozen and slushy, about 2 hours.

Sunday

Breakfast

Breakfast-Granola Parfait

Use any fruit that is fresh, ripe, and in season. In the summer try peaches and apricots. In the fall, try ripe, juicy pears and pomegranate seeds. Winter is citrus season, so look for fancy tangerines, mandarins, and blood oranges.

1. Put ½ cup of fruit in the bottom of each parfait glass. Layer ¼ cup of yogurt over the fruit, then ¼ cup granola. Repeat the layering, finishing with the granola on top.

2. Before serving, drizzle one tablespoon of honey on top of each glass, and garnish with a whole fresh berry, or wedge of fruit.

Lunch

Grilled Tuna Niçoise

See recipe, Chapter 6.

Snack

Whole-Wheat Baguette with Roquefort Spread

Bread flour can be found in any supermarket. You can also find whole-grain bread flour at health food stores.

1. In a medium bowl, combine water, yeast, and honey and let stand 10 minutes. Add whole-wheat flour and salt and combine thoroughly. Slowly add enough bread flour to create a firm dough. Turn out onto floured surface and knead, adding flour only as necessary, until it becomes smooth and elastic, about 8–10 minutes. Return to the bowl, cover with plastic wrap, and set in a warm place to rise until doubled in volume, about 1 hour.

2. Coat a baking sheet with pan spray and sprinkle with cornmeal. Turn dough out onto a floured surface and divide into 3 equal portions. Roll each piece into a tight rope and taper the ends slightly. Place loaves on pan, dust with flour, cover with plastic wrap, and rise another 30 minutes. Preheat oven to 400°F.

3. Score ¼-inch-deep angled cuts in the top of each loaf, to allow dough to expand decoratively during baking. Bake until golden brown and firm, about 15–20 minutes. Cool completely before slicing and serving with softened cheese.

Dinner

Celery Root Remoulade

Look for celery root in the fall and winter, sometimes under the name celeriac. It looks like a wide, knobby potato and has a carrot-like texture and a subtle, celery flavor.

In a large bowl, whisk together lemon, oil, mustard, vinegar, herbs, and pepper. Add celery root and toss to coat. Cover and marinate 30 minutes before serving.

Whole-Wheat Baguette with Roquefort Spread
MAKES 3 (18-INCH) LOAVES

INGREDIENTS
2 cups warm water
2 (.25-ounce) packages active dry yeast
1 tablespoon honey
2 cups whole-wheat flour
1 teaspoon kosher salt
3 cups bread flour
¼ cup cornmeal
¼ pound Roquefort cheese, room temperature

Celery Root Remoulade
SERVES 4–6

INGREDIENTS
2 tablespoons lemon juice
⅓ cup olive oil
1 tablespoon Dijon mustard
2 teaspoons white wine vinegar
1 tablespoon chopped chervil or tarragon
1 teaspoon black pepper
1 pound celery root, peeled and grated

Whole-Wheat Orange Crepes

See Raspberry Crepes recipe, Chapter 16. Replace raspberries and raspberry jam with orange slices and orange marmalade.

Dijon-Marinated Grilled Chicken

You can cook this dish under a broiler, too. Turn it often to promote even browning.

1. In a small bowl combine lemon zest and juice, salt, pepper, paprika, thyme, rosemary, tarragon, scallions, garlic, ½ cup oil, and mustard. Place chicken in a large zipper bag, and add marinade. Zip it tight and massage marinade into the chicken. Refrigerate for 1 hour or overnight.

2. Preheat grill on high heat. Grill skin side down over direct high heat for 5 minutes with the lid down. Reduce heat to low, flip chicken over and move off direct heat. Close cover and cook for 45–60 minutes, basting with marinade every 10 minutes as needed.

Appendix B
Good Sources of Nutrients

Good Sources of Vitamin A

Apricot

Broccoli

Cantaloupe

Carrots

Collards

Kale

Mango

Pumpkin

Spinach

Squash, winter

Sweet potato

Tomato

Turnip greens

Watermelon

Good Sources of Vitamin C

Apple with skin

Apricot, dried

Banana

Beans, lima

Broccoli

Cantaloupe

Collards

Grapefruit

Grapefruit juice

Honeydew melon

Kale

Kiwi

Orange

Orange juice

Pear with skin

Peas, green

Peppers

Potato, with skin

Spinach

Squash, winter

Strawberries

Sweet Potato

Tomato

Turnip greens

Watermelon

Good Sources of Folate

Beans,dry

Black-eyed Peas

Broccoli

Lentils

Mustard greens

Orange

Orange juice

Peas, green

Peas, split

Spinach

Turnip greens

Good Sources of Potassium

Apricots, dried

Banana

Beans, dry

Black-eyed peas

Cantaloupe

Grapefruit juice

Honeydew melon

Lentils

Orange juice

Peas, green

Peas, split

Plantains

Potato with skin

Prune juice

Spinach, cooked

Squash, winter

Sweet potato

Tomato

Good Sources of Dietary Fiber

Apple with skin

Apricot,dried

Banana

Beans, dry

Beans, lima

Black-eyed peas

Broccoli

Carrots

Lentils

Orange

Pear with skin

Peas, green

Peas, split

Potato with skin

Prunes

Spinach

Squash, winter

Strawberries

Sweet potato

Body Mass Index (BMI) Table

BMI	19	20	21	22	23	24	25	26	27	28	29	30	31	32	33	34	35	36	37	38	39	40	41	42	43	44	45	46	47	48	49	50	51	52	53	54
Height (inches)												Body weight (pounds)																								
58	91	96	100	105	110	115	119	124	129	134	138	143	148	153	158	162	167	172	177	181	186	191	196	201	205	210	215	220	224	229	234	239	244	248	253	258
59	94	99	104	109	114	119	124	128	133	138	143	148	153	158	163	168	173	178	183	188	193	198	203	208	212	217	222	227	232	237	242	247	252	257	262	267
60	97	102	107	112	118	123	128	133	138	143	148	153	158	163	168	174	179	184	189	194	199	204	209	215	220	225	230	235	240	245	250	255	261	266	271	276
61	100	106	111	116	122	127	132	137	143	148	153	158	164	169	174	180	185	190	195	201	206	211	217	222	227	232	238	243	248	254	259	264	269	275	280	285
62	104	109	115	120	126	131	136	142	147	153	158	164	169	175	180	186	191	196	202	207	213	218	224	229	235	240	246	251	256	262	267	273	278	284	289	295
63	107	113	118	124	130	135	141	146	152	158	163	169	175	180	186	191	197	203	208	214	220	225	231	237	242	248	254	259	265	270	278	282	287	293	299	304
64	110	116	122	128	134	140	145	151	157	163	169	174	180	186	192	197	204	209	215	221	227	232	238	244	250	256	262	267	273	279	285	291	296	302	308	314
65	114	120	126	132	138	144	150	156	162	168	174	180	186	192	198	204	210	216	222	228	234	240	246	252	258	264	270	276	282	288	294	300	306	312	318	324
66	118	124	130	136	142	148	155	161	167	173	179	186	192	198	204	210	216	223	229	235	241	247	253	260	266	272	278	284	291	297	303	309	315	322	328	334
67	121	127	134	140	146	153	159	166	172	178	185	191	198	204	211	217	223	230	236	242	249	255	261	268	274	280	287	293	299	306	312	319	325	331	338	344
68	125	131	138	144	151	158	164	171	177	184	190	197	203	210	216	223	230	236	243	249	256	262	269	276	282	289	295	302	308	315	322	328	335	341	348	354
69	128	135	142	149	155	162	169	176	182	189	196	203	209	216	223	230	236	243	250	257	263	270	277	284	291	297	304	311	318	324	331	338	345	351	358	365
70	132	139	146	153	160	167	174	181	188	195	202	209	216	222	229	236	243	250	257	264	271	278	285	292	299	306	313	320	327	334	341	348	355	362	369	376
71	136	143	150	157	165	172	179	186	193	200	208	215	222	229	236	243	250	257	265	272	279	286	293	301	308	315	322	329	338	343	351	358	365	372	379	386
72	140	147	154	162	169	177	184	191	199	206	213	221	228	235	242	250	258	265	272	279	287	294	302	309	316	324	331	338	346	353	361	368	375	383	390	397
73	144	151	159	166	174	182	189	197	204	212	219	227	235	242	250	257	265	272	280	288	295	302	310	318	325	333	340	348	355	363	371	378	386	393	401	408
74	148	155	163	171	179	186	194	202	210	218	225	233	241	249	256	264	272	280	287	295	303	311	319	326	334	342	350	358	365	373	381	389	396	404	412	420
75	152	160	168	176	184	192	200	208	216	224	232	240	248	256	264	272	279	287	295	303	311	319	327	335	343	351	359	367	375	383	391	399	407	415	423	431
76	156	164	172	180	189	197	205	213	221	230	238	246	254	263	271	279	287	295	304	312	320	328	336	344	353	361	369	377	385	394	402	410	418	426	435	443

Normal **Overweight** **Obese** **Extreme Obesity**

Source: Adapted from *Clinical Guidelines on the Identification, Evaluation, and Treatment of Overweight and Obesity in Adults: The Evidence Report.*

Appendix D
Glossary

al dente
An Italian term that means "to the tooth," and refers to the degree to which certain foods, usually pasta and vegetables, are cooked. These foods are cooked until done, but still have slight texture when bitten. They are not raw, or crunchy, nor are they soft.

antioxidants
Molecules that slow oxidation of other molecules. Oxidation can produce free radicals, which trigger chain reactions that damage cells. In addition to preventing these reactions, antioxidants can inhibit them once begun.

baste
To coat food with fat or liquid as it cooks in order to preserve moisture. A bulb baster is a suction-based tool.

blanch
To boil briefly then submerge in ice water to halt cooking. The process is used to loosen skin and intensify the color of vegetables and fruits. Also referred to as parboiling.

botulism
A potentially fatal food-borne illness, caused by ingestion of the nerve toxin botulin, most commonly occurring from improperly canned foods.

capers
Small buds from an evergreen shrub, pickled in salty, vinegar-based brine.

caramelized
To cook food until the sugar, naturally occurring or added, darkens to an amber "caramel" color. Caramelizing brings out the food's deep, sweet, rich flavors.

celery root
The edible, bulbous root of the celery plant. Also known as celeriac.

cheesecloth
A fine linen mesh cloth, traditionally used in cheese making to strain whey from curds. Used by chefs for fine straining of all foods, as well as a covering, wrapping, or steeping foods.

chutney
A chunky condiment from Southern Asia and India, sometimes cooked and jam-like, made with fruits or vegetables and often spiced with chilies.

currants
These tiny raisins are made from dried miniature seedless grapes.

curry powder
A spice blend originated by the British during their colonial rule of India so they could bring home the flavor of the regional curry dishes. The flavor of the powder found in supermarkets is fairly generic, but throughout India and other parts of Asia, there are dozens of unique curry sauce variations.

daily value

This percentage is the recommended daily intake of key nutrients based on a 2,000-calorie diet. Its listing on food labels is meant as a guide to help determine the relative nutritional value of foods.

diuretic

A drug that increases the body's excretion of water through urine. The most common household diuretic is caffeine.

E. coli

A bacterium (*Escherichia coli*) that is naturally occurring in the human intestinal tract, but certain strains can cause serious gastrointestinal distress and, in some cases, death. It is most commonly caused by under-cooked meats and cross-contamination.

electrolytes

This is the scientific name for electrically charged salt ions. They are what your cells use to maintain and conduct electric impulses. Kidneys help to maintain electrolyte balance, but through sweat and other body fluid loss, electrolytes are lost as well. Several beverages on the market, including sports drinks, contain added electrolytes.

empty calories

This term denotes foods that contain calories but no viable nutrients. The category encompasses all "junk" foods.

fish sauce

A liquid condiment and ingredient similar in appearance to soy sauce, made from fermented fish. Popular in Asia, fish sauce was known in ancient Rome.

garam masala

The most common spice blend from Northern India. The word *garam* means "warm," or "hot," and while it can be spicy, the name denotes the toasting of the spices prior to grinding.

garum

The ancient Roman name for fish sauce, a condiment made from fermented, aged fish. Similar sauces are still made and used today throughout Asia.

gluten

A protein in flour that, when moistened and agitated, becomes firm and elastic. This effect traps the gasses of fermentation, which allows dough to rise.

Gorgonzola

Commonly referred to as a blue-vein cheese, this Italian cow's milk cheese has veins that appear more green than blue. Made since the Middle Ages, Gorgonzola can be creamy, crumbly, or firm. Its piquant flavor comes from the addition of bacteria, added and allowed to germinate into mold.

Gruyere

A nutty, semifirm cow's milk cheese from Switzerland.

herbes de Provence

A spice and herb blend commonly used in Mediterranean cuisine, including lavender, thyme, sage, marjoram, basil, rosemary, fennel, and savory.

hydrogenated

Unsaturated fat (vegetable based) that is artificially saturated by the introduction of hydrogen.

infuse

To steep two foods or flavors together.

injera
A spongy, pancake-like Ethiopian bread, used as a utensil to scoop up the traditional spicy stews.

Italian seasoning
A spice and herb blend commonly used in Italian recipes, including fennel, rosemary, basil, and oregano.

jicima
A sweet, crisp tuber, with white flesh and thin brown papery skin, usually eaten raw.

julienne
A classic knife cut that looks like long, thick matchsticks.

kalamata
Greek black olives marinated in wine and olive oil.

legume
A plant with long seed pods containing beans or seeds, such as lentils, peanuts, and soybeans.

macerate
To soak food, usually fruit, in liquid to infuse flavor.

madras
A mild to hot red curry sauce from India.

millet
A tiny, bland grain packed with protein, which can be boiled like rice or ground into flour.

mortar
A bowl, usually made of ceramic or stone, in which spices, herbs, or vegetables are crushed by a pestle, a hard instrument shaped like a small baseball bat.

nutrient-dense
This term refers to foods that are rich in nutrients but low in calories. Nutrient-dense foods in general are considered the opposite of "empty calories."

polenta
Cornmeal mush from Northern Italy.

pulse
The dried seeds of legumes.

puree
Any food pulverized to a smooth paste of varying consistencies.

quinoa
An ancient Incan grain, and one of the few vegetable sources of complete protein.

rancid
Oxidation of oil that results in foul flavor and odor.

raw cuisine
The promotion of the consumption of uncooked, unprocessed, and usually organic foods. It is generally believed that consumption of raw foods can prevent and heal many forms of sickness and chronic disease. Also known as raw foodism.

reduce
A culinary term meaning to cook the water out of a dish, reducing its volume, intensifying its flavor, and thickening its consistency.

Roquefort
A French blue cheese made specifically from sheep's milk, exposed to Penicillium roqueforte mold spores, and aged in limestone caves in southwestern France.

rotini
An Italian pasta shaped like a corkscrew.

roux
A thickening agent made with equal parts melted fat (usually butter) and flour.

sake
A Japanese rice wine.

sauté
To cook food quickly, over high heat, constantly stirring for even browning. The term comes from the French for "to jump," and sauté pans are designed with a curved lip, making constant motion as easy as a flick of the wrist.

sear
To brown food, usually meat, on all sides at very high temperature, ostensibly to seal in the meat's juice. The ability to retain the liquid in food by this method is under some scrutiny.

seize
A term that refers to the thickening and hardening of melted chocolate that occurs when a small amount of moisture is added.

star anise
A potent anise-flavored spice from a star-shaped fruit from an evergreen tree.

tahini
A paste made of ground sesame seeds.

tortilla
A Spanish word with several meanings; it refers to flat bread in Mexico and an open-faced omelet in Spain.

zest
The colorful outermost rind of a citrus fruit, containing a high concentration of the essential oils and flavor compounds that flavor the fruit itself.

Index

THE EVERYTHING SERIES!

BUSINESS & PERSONAL FINANCE

Everything® Accounting Book
Everything® Budgeting Book, 2nd Ed.
Everything® Business Planning Book
Everything® Coaching and Mentoring Book, 2nd Ed.
Everything® Fundraising Book
Everything® Get Out of Debt Book
Everything® Grant Writing Book, 2nd Ed.
Everything® Guide to Buying Foreclosures
Everything® Guide to Fundraising, $15.95
Everything® Guide to Mortgages
Everything® Guide to Personal Finance for Single Mothers
Everything® Home-Based Business Book, 2nd Ed.
Everything® Homebuying Book, 3rd Ed., $15.95
Everything® Homeselling Book, 2nd Ed.
Everything® Human Resource Management Book
Everything® Improve Your Credit Book
Everything® Investing Book, 2nd Ed.
Everything® Landlording Book
Everything® Leadership Book, 2nd Ed.
Everything® Managing People Book, 2nd Ed.
Everything® Negotiating Book
Everything® Online Auctions Book
Everything® Online Business Book
Everything® Personal Finance Book
Everything® Personal Finance in Your 20s & 30s Book, 2nd Ed.
Everything® Personal Finance in Your 40s & 50s Book, $15.95
Everything® Project Management Book, 2nd Ed.
Everything® Real Estate Investing Book
Everything® Retirement Planning Book
Everything® Robert's Rules Book, $7.95
Everything® Selling Book
Everything® Start Your Own Business Book, 2nd Ed.
Everything® Wills & Estate Planning Book

COOKING

Everything® Barbecue Cookbook
Everything® Bartender's Book, 2nd Ed., $9.95
Everything® Calorie Counting Cookbook
Everything® Cheese Book
Everything® Chinese Cookbook
Everything® Classic Recipes Book
Everything® Cocktail Parties & Drinks Book
Everything® College Cookbook
Everything® Cooking for Baby and Toddler Book
Everything® Diabetes Cookbook
Everything® Easy Gourmet Cookbook
Everything® Fondue Cookbook
Everything® Food Allergy Cookbook, $15.95
Everything® Fondue Party Book
Everything® Gluten-Free Cookbook
Everything® Glycemic Index Cookbook
Everything® Grilling Cookbook
Everything® Healthy Cooking for Parties Book, $15.95
Everything® Holiday Cookbook
Everything® Indian Cookbook
Everything® Lactose-Free Cookbook
Everything® Low-Cholesterol Cookbook

Everything® Low-Fat High-Flavor Cookbook, 2nd Ed., $15.95
Everything® Low-Salt Cookbook
Everything® Meals for a Month Cookbook
Everything® Meals on a Budget Cookbook
Everything® Mediterranean Cookbook
Everything® Mexican Cookbook
Everything® No Trans Fat Cookbook
Everything® One-Pot Cookbook, 2nd Ed., $15.95
Everything® Organic Cooking for Baby & Toddler Book, $15.95
Everything® Pizza Cookbook
Everything® Quick Meals Cookbook, 2nd Ed., $15.95
Everything® Slow Cooker Cookbook
Everything® Slow Cooking for a Crowd Cookbook
Everything® Soup Cookbook
Everything® Stir-Fry Cookbook
Everything® Sugar-Free Cookbook
Everything® Tapas and Small Plates Cookbook
Everything® Tex-Mex Cookbook
Everything® Thai Cookbook
Everything® Vegetarian Cookbook
Everything® Whole-Grain, High-Fiber Cookbook
Everything® Wild Game Cookbook
Everything® Wine Book, 2nd Ed.

GAMES

Everything® 15-Minute Sudoku Book, $9.95
Everything® 30-Minute Sudoku Book, $9.95
Everything® Bible Crosswords Book, $9.95
Everything® Blackjack Strategy Book
Everything® Brain Strain Book, $9.95
Everything® Bridge Book
Everything® Card Games Book
Everything® Card Tricks Book, $9.95
Everything® Casino Gambling Book, 2nd Ed.
Everything® Chess Basics Book
Everything® Christmas Crosswords Book, $9.95
Everything® Craps Strategy Book
Everything® Crossword and Puzzle Book
Everything® Crosswords and Puzzles for Quote Lovers Book, $9.95
Everything® Crossword Challenge Book
Everything® Crosswords for the Beach Book, $9.95
Everything® Cryptic Crosswords Book, $9.95
Everything® Cryptograms Book, $9.95
Everything® Easy Crosswords Book
Everything® Easy Kakuro Book, $9.95
Everything® Easy Large-Print Crosswords Book
Everything® Games Book, 2nd Ed.
Everything® Giant Book of Crosswords
Everything® Giant Sudoku Book, $9.95
Everything® Giant Word Search Book
Everything® Kakuro Challenge Book, $9.95
Everything® Large-Print Crossword Challenge Book
Everything® Large-Print Crosswords Book
Everything® Large-Print Travel Crosswords Book
Everything® Lateral Thinking Puzzles Book, $9.95
Everything® Literary Crosswords Book, $9.95
Everything® Mazes Book
Everything® Memory Booster Puzzles Book, $9.95

Everything® Movie Crosswords Book, $9.95
Everything® Music Crosswords Book, $9.95
Everything® Online Poker Book
Everything® Pencil Puzzles Book, $9.95
Everything® Poker Strategy Book
Everything® Pool & Billiards Book
Everything® Puzzles for Commuters Book, $9.95
Everything® Puzzles for Dog Lovers Book, $9.95
Everything® Sports Crosswords Book, $9.95
Everything® Test Your IQ Book, $9.95
Everything® Texas Hold 'Em Book, $9.95
Everything® Travel Crosswords Book, $9.95
Everything® Travel Mazes Book, $9.95
Everything® Travel Word Search Book, $9.95
Everything® TV Crosswords Book, $9.95
Everything® Word Games Challenge Book
Everything® Word Scramble Book
Everything® Word Search Book

HEALTH

Everything® Alzheimer's Book
Everything® Diabetes Book
Everything® First Aid Book, $9.95
Everything® Green Living Book
Everything® Health Guide to Addiction and Recovery
Everything® Health Guide to Adult Bipolar Disorder
Everything® Health Guide to Arthritis
Everything® Health Guide to Controlling Anxiety
Everything® Health Guide to Depression
Everything® Health Guide to Diabetes, 2nd Ed.
Everything® Health Guide to Fibromyalgia
Everything® Health Guide to Menopause, 2nd Ed.
Everything® Health Guide to Migraines
Everything® Health Guide to Multiple Sclerosis
Everything® Health Guide to OCD
Everything® Health Guide to PMS
Everything® Health Guide to Postpartum Care
Everything® Health Guide to Thyroid Disease
Everything® Hypnosis Book
Everything® Low Cholesterol Book
Everything® Menopause Book
Everything® Nutrition Book
Everything® Reflexology Book
Everything® Stress Management Book
Everything® Superfoods Book, $15.95

HISTORY

Everything® American Government Book
Everything® American History Book, 2nd Ed.
Everything® American Revolution Book, $15.95
Everything® Civil War Book
Everything® Freemasons Book
Everything® Irish History & Heritage Book
Everything® World War II Book, 2nd Ed.

HOBBIES

Everything® Candlemaking Book
Everything® Cartooning Book
Everything® Coin Collecting Book
Everything® Digital Photography Book, 2nd Ed.

Everything® Drawing Book
Everything® Family Tree Book, 2nd Ed.
Everything® Guide to Online Genealogy, $15.95
Everything® Knitting Book
Everything® Knots Book
Everything® Photography Book
Everything® Quilting Book
Everything® Sewing Book
Everything® Soapmaking Book, 2nd Ed.
Everything® Woodworking Book

HOME IMPROVEMENT

Everything® Feng Shui Book
Everything® Feng Shui Decluttering Book, $9.95
Everything® Fix-It Book
Everything® Green Living Book
Everything® Home Decorating Book
Everything® Home Storage Solutions Book
Everything® Homebuilding Book
Everything® Organize Your Home Book, 2nd Ed.

KIDS' BOOKS

All titles are $7.95

Everything® Fairy Tales Book, $14.95
Everything® Kids' Animal Puzzle & Activity Book
Everything® Kids' Astronomy Book
Everything® Kids' Baseball Book, 5th Ed.
Everything® Kids' Bible Trivia Book
Everything® Kids' Bugs Book
Everything® Kids' Cars and Trucks Puzzle and Activity Book
Everything® Kids' Christmas Puzzle & Activity Book
Everything® Kids' Connect the Dots
    Puzzle and Activity Book
Everything® Kids' Cookbook, 2nd Ed.
Everything® Kids' Crazy Puzzles Book
Everything® Kids' Dinosaurs Book
Everything® Kids' Dragons Puzzle and Activity Book
Everything® Kids' Environment Book $7.95
Everything® Kids' Fairies Puzzle and Activity Book
Everything® Kids' First Spanish Puzzle and Activity Book
Everything® Kids' Football Book
Everything® Kids' Geography Book
Everything® Kids' Gross Cookbook
Everything® Kids' Gross Hidden Pictures Book
Everything® Kids' Gross Jokes Book
Everything® Kids' Gross Mazes Book
Everything® Kids' Gross Puzzle & Activity Book
Everything® Kids' Halloween Puzzle & Activity Book
Everything® Kids' Hanukkah Puzzle and Activity Book
Everything® Kids' Hidden Pictures Book
Everything® Kids' Horses Book
Everything® Kids' Joke Book
Everything® Kids' Knock Knock Book
Everything® Kids' Learning French Book
Everything® Kids' Learning Spanish Book
Everything® Kids' Magical Science Experiments Book
Everything® Kids' Math Puzzles Book
Everything® Kids' Mazes Book
Everything® Kids' Money Book, 2nd Ed.
Everything® Kids' Mummies, Pharaoh's, and Pyramids
    Puzzle and Activity Book
Everything® Kids' Nature Book
Everything® Kids' Pirates Puzzle and Activity Book
Everything® Kids' Presidents Book
Everything® Kids' Princess Puzzle and Activity Book
Everything® Kids' Puzzle Book

Everything® Kids' Racecars Puzzle and Activity Book
Everything® Kids' Riddles & Brain Teasers Book
Everything® Kids' Science Experiments Book
Everything® Kids' Sharks Book
Everything® Kids' Soccer Book
Everything® Kids' Spelling Book
Everything® Kids' Spies Puzzle and Activity Book
Everything® Kids' States Book
Everything® Kids' Travel Activity Book
Everything® Kids' Word Search Puzzle and Activity Book

LANGUAGE

Everything® Conversational Japanese Book with CD, $19.95
Everything® French Grammar Book
Everything® French Phrase Book, $9.95
Everything® French Verb Book, $9.95
Everything® German Phrase Book, $9.95
Everything® German Practice Book with CD, $19.95
Everything® Inglés Book
Everything® Intermediate Spanish Book with CD, $19.95
Everything® Italian Phrase Book, $9.95
Everything® Italian Practice Book with CD, $19.95
Everything® Learning Brazilian Portuguese Book with CD, $19.95
Everything® Learning French Book with CD, 2nd Ed., $19.95
Everything® Learning German Book
Everything® Learning Italian Book
Everything® Learning Latin Book
Everything® Learning Russian Book with CD, $19.95
Everything® Learning Spanish Book
Everything® Learning Spanish Book with CD, 2nd Ed., $19.95
Everything® Russian Practice Book with CD, $19.95
Everything® Sign Language Book, $15.95
Everything® Spanish Grammar Book
Everything® Spanish Phrase Book, $9.95
Everything® Spanish Practice Book with CD, $19.95
Everything® Spanish Verb Book, $9.95
Everything® Speaking Mandarin Chinese Book with CD, $19.95

MUSIC

Everything® Bass Guitar Book with CD, $19.95
Everything® Drums Book with CD, $19.95
Everything® Guitar Book with CD, 2nd Ed., $19.95
Everything® Guitar Chords Book with CD, $19.95
Everything® Guitar Scales Book with CD, $19.95
Everything® Harmonica Book with CD, $15.95
Everything® Home Recording Book
Everything® Music Theory Book with CD, $19.95
Everything® Reading Music Book with CD, $19.95
Everything® Rock & Blues Guitar Book with CD, $19.95
Everything® Rock & Blues Piano Book with CD, $19.95
Everything® Rock Drums Book with CD, $19.95
Everything® Singing Book with CD, $19.95
Everything® Songwriting Book

NEW AGE

Everything® Astrology Book, 2nd Ed.
Everything® Birthday Personology Book
Everything® Celtic Wisdom Book, $15.95
Everything® Dreams Book, 2nd Ed.
Everything® Law of Attraction Book, $15.95
Everything® Love Signs Book, $9.95
Everything® Love Spells Book, $9.95
Everything® Palmistry Book
Everything® Psychic Book
Everything® Reiki Book

Everything® Sex Signs Book, $9.95
Everything® Spells & Charms Book, 2nd Ed.
Everything® Tarot Book, 2nd Ed.
Everything® Toltec Wisdom Book
Everything® Wicca & Witchcraft Book, 2nd Ed.

PARENTING

Everything® Baby Names Book, 2nd Ed.
Everything® Baby Shower Book, 2nd Ed.
Everything® Baby Sign Language Book with DVD
Everything® Baby's First Year Book
Everything® Birthing Book
Everything® Breastfeeding Book
Everything® Father-to-Be Book
Everything® Father's First Year Book
Everything® Get Ready for Baby Book, 2nd Ed.
Everything® Get Your Baby to Sleep Book, $9.95
Everything® Getting Pregnant Book
Everything® Guide to Pregnancy Over 35
Everything® Guide to Raising a One-Year-Old
Everything® Guide to Raising a Two-Year-Old
Everything® Guide to Raising Adolescent Boys
Everything® Guide to Raising Adolescent Girls
Everything® Mother's First Year Book
Everything® Parent's Guide to Childhood Illnesses
Everything® Parent's Guide to Children and Divorce
Everything® Parent's Guide to Children with ADD/ADHD
Everything® Parent's Guide to Children with Asperger's
    Syndrome
Everything® Parent's Guide to Children with Anxiety
Everything® Parent's Guide to Children with Asthma
Everything® Parent's Guide to Children with Autism
Everything® Parent's Guide to Children with Bipolar Disorder
Everything® Parent's Guide to Children with Depression
Everything® Parent's Guide to Children with Dyslexia
Everything® Parent's Guide to Children with Juvenile Diabetes
Everything® Parent's Guide to Children with OCD
Everything® Parent's Guide to Positive Discipline
Everything® Parent's Guide to Raising Boys
Everything® Parent's Guide to Raising Girls
Everything® Parent's Guide to Raising Siblings
Everything® Parent's Guide to Raising Your
    Adopted Child
Everything® Parent's Guide to Sensory Integration Disorder
Everything® Parent's Guide to Tantrums
Everything® Parent's Guide to the Strong-Willed Child
Everything® Parenting a Teenager Book
Everything® Potty Training Book, $9.95
Everything® Pregnancy Book, 3rd Ed.
Everything® Pregnancy Fitness Book
Everything® Pregnancy Nutrition Book
Everything® Pregnancy Organizer, 2nd Ed., $16.95
Everything® Toddler Activities Book
Everything® Toddler Book
Everything® Tween Book
Everything® Twins, Triplets, and More Book

PETS

Everything® Aquarium Book
Everything® Boxer Book
Everything® Cat Book, 2nd Ed.
Everything® Chihuahua Book
Everything® Cooking for Dogs Book
Everything® Dachshund Book
Everything® Dog Book, 2nd Ed.
Everything® Dog Grooming Book

Everything® Dog Obedience Book
Everything® Dog Owner's Organizer, $16.95
Everything® Dog Training and Tricks Book
Everything® German Shepherd Book
Everything® Golden Retriever Book
Everything® Horse Book, 2nd Ed., $15.95
Everything® Horse Care Book
Everything® Horseback Riding Book
Everything® Labrador Retriever Book
Everything® Poodle Book
Everything® Pug Book
Everything® Puppy Book
Everything® Small Dogs Book
Everything® Tropical Fish Book
Everything® Yorkshire Terrier Book

REFERENCE

Everything® American Presidents Book
Everything® Blogging Book
Everything® Build Your Vocabulary Book, $9.95
Everything® Car Care Book
Everything® Classical Mythology Book
Everything® Da Vinci Book
Everything® Einstein Book
Everything® Enneagram Book
Everything® Etiquette Book, 2nd Ed.
Everything® Family Christmas Book, $15.95
Everything® Guide to C. S. Lewis & Narnia
Everything® Guide to Divorce, 2nd Ed., $15.95
Everything® Guide to Edgar Allan Poe
Everything® Guide to Understanding Philosophy
Everything® Inventions and Patents Book
Everything® Jacqueline Kennedy Onassis Book
Everything® John F. Kennedy Book
Everything® Mafia Book
Everything® Martin Luther King Jr. Book
Everything® Pirates Book
Everything® Private Investigation Book
Everything® Psychology Book
Everything® Public Speaking Book, $9.95
Everything® Shakespeare Book, 2nd Ed.

RELIGION

Everything® Angels Book
Everything® Bible Book
Everything® Bible Study Book with CD, $19.95
Everything® Buddhism Book
Everything® Catholicism Book
Everything® Christianity Book
Everything® Gnostic Gospels Book
Everything® Hinduism Book, $15.95
Everything® History of the Bible Book
Everything® Jesus Book
Everything® Jewish History & Heritage Book
Everything® Judaism Book
Everything® Kabbalah Book
Everything® Koran Book
Everything® Mary Book
Everything® Mary Magdalene Book
Everything® Prayer Book

Everything® Saints Book, 2nd Ed.
Everything® Torah Book
Everything® Understanding Islam Book
Everything® Women of the Bible Book
Everything® World's Religions Book

SCHOOL & CAREERS

Everything® Career Tests Book
Everything® College Major Test Book
Everything® College Survival Book, 2nd Ed.
Everything® Cover Letter Book, 2nd Ed.
Everything® Filmmaking Book
Everything® Get-a-Job Book, 2nd Ed.
Everything® Guide to Being a Paralegal
Everything® Guide to Being a Personal Trainer
Everything® Guide to Being a Real Estate Agent
Everything® Guide to Being a Sales Rep
Everything® Guide to Being an Event Planner
Everything® Guide to Careers in Health Care
Everything® Guide to Careers in Law Enforcement
Everything® Guide to Government Jobs
Everything® Guide to Starting and Running a Catering
    Business
Everything® Guide to Starting and Running a Restaurant
**Everything® Guide to Starting and Running
    a Retail Store**
Everything® Job Interview Book, 2nd Ed.
Everything® New Nurse Book
Everything® New Teacher Book
Everything® Paying for College Book
Everything® Practice Interview Book
Everything® Resume Book, 3rd Ed.
Everything® Study Book

SELF-HELP

Everything® Body Language Book
Everything® Dating Book, 2nd Ed.
Everything® Great Sex Book
**Everything® Guide to Caring for Aging Parents,
    $15.95**
Everything® Self-Esteem Book
Everything® Self-Hypnosis Book, $9.95
Everything® Tantric Sex Book

SPORTS & FITNESS

Everything® Easy Fitness Book
Everything® Fishing Book
Everything® Guide to Weight Training, $15.95
Everything® Krav Maga for Fitness Book
Everything® Running Book, 2nd Ed.
Everything® Triathlon Training Book, $15.95

TRAVEL

Everything® Family Guide to Coastal Florida
Everything® Family Guide to Cruise Vacations
Everything® Family Guide to Hawaii
Everything® Family Guide to Las Vegas, 2nd Ed.
Everything® Family Guide to Mexico
Everything® Family Guide to New England, 2nd Ed.

Everything® Family Guide to New York City, 3rd Ed.
**Everything® Family Guide to Northern California
    and Lake Tahoe**
Everything® Family Guide to RV Travel & Campgrounds
Everything® Family Guide to the Caribbean
Everything® Family Guide to the Disneyland® Resort, California
    Adventure®, Universal Studios®, and the Anaheim
    Area, 2nd Ed.
Everything® Family Guide to the Walt Disney World Resort®,
    Universal Studios®, and Greater Orlando, 5th Ed.
Everything® Family Guide to Timeshares
Everything® Family Guide to Washington D.C., 2nd Ed.

WEDDINGS

Everything® Bachelorette Party Book, $9.95
Everything® Bridesmaid Book, $9.95
Everything® Destination Wedding Book
Everything® Father of the Bride Book, $9.95
Everything® Green Wedding Book, $15.95
Everything® Groom Book, $9.95
Everything® Jewish Wedding Book, 2nd Ed., $15.95
Everything® Mother of the Bride Book, $9.95
Everything® Outdoor Wedding Book
Everything® Wedding Book, 3rd Ed.
Everything® Wedding Checklist, $9.95
Everything® Wedding Etiquette Book, $9.95
Everything® Wedding Organizer, 2nd Ed., $16.95
Everything® Wedding Shower Book, $9.95
Everything® Wedding Vows Book, 3rd Ed., $9.95
Everything® Wedding Workout Book
Everything® Weddings on a Budget Book, 2nd Ed., $9.95

WRITING

Everything® Creative Writing Book
Everything® Get Published Book, 2nd Ed.
Everything® Grammar and Style Book, 2nd Ed.
Everything® Guide to Magazine Writing
Everything® Guide to Writing a Book Proposal
Everything® Guide to Writing a Novel
Everything® Guide to Writing Children's Books
Everything® Guide to Writing Copy
Everything® Guide to Writing Graphic Novels
Everything® Guide to Writing Research Papers
Everything® Guide to Writing a Romance Novel, $15.95
Everything® Improve Your Writing Book, 2nd Ed.
Everything® Writing Poetry Book